THE EMERGENCY DEPARTMENT
A SURVIVAL GUIDE

THE EMERGENCY DEPARTMENT
A SURVIVAL GUIDE

Jon Whittaker
MBChB DA FRCS (Edin) FFAEM
Consultant in Emergency Medicine
Lancashire Teaching Hospitals NHS Trust
Preston

Anne Brickwood
BSc MBChB
Senior House Officer
Critical Care Rotation
Whiston Hospital
Merseyside

Andrew Curran
BSc MBChB MRCS A&E (Edin) DIMC
Specialist Registrar in Emergency Medicine
North West England Deanery

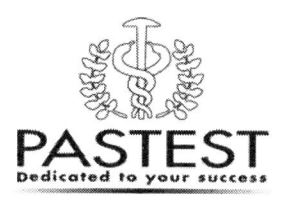

PASTEST
Dedicated to your success

© 2004 PASTEST Ltd
Egerton Court
Parkgate Estate
Knutsford
Cheshire
WA16 8DX

Telephone: 01565 752000

All rights reserved. No part of this publication may be reproduced, stored in a retrieval system, or transmitted, in any form or by any means, electronic, mechanical, photocopying, recording or otherwise, without the prior permission of the copyright owner.

First published 2004

Reprinted 2007

ISBN: 1 901198 21 9
ISBN: 978 1 901198 21 8

A catalogue record for this book is available from the British Library.

The information contained within this book was obtained by the authors from reliable sources. However, while every effort has been made to ensure its accuracy, no responsibility for loss, damage or injury occasioned to any person acting or refraining from action as a result of information contained herein can be accepted by the publishers or authors.

PasTest Revision Books and Intensive Courses

PasTest has been established in the field of postgraduate medical education since 1972, providing revision books and intensive study courses for doctors preparing for their professional examinations. Books and courses are available for the following specialties:

MRCGP, MRCP Part 1 and 2, MRCPCH Part 1 and 2, MRCPsych, MRCS, MRCOG, DRCOG, DCH, FRCA, PLAB.

For further details contact:

PasTest, Freepost, Knutsford, Cheshire WA16 7BR
Tel: 01565 752000 Fax: 01565 650264
www.pastest.co.uk   enquiries@pastest.co.uk

Text prepared by Vision Typesetting Ltd, Manchester
Printed and bound in Great Britain by
Athenaeum Press, Gateshead

CONTENTS

PREFACE *page* vii
INTRODUCTION ix
  How to use this book ix
  Risks and difficulties of working in the emergency
    department xi
  Giving pain relief xiii
  Abbreviations xv
  Table of normal haematological and biochemical
    values xvii

Part A: ILLNESS 1

Chapter 1: MEDICAL 3
Cardiac arrest 4
  Cardiac arrest flowchart 4
Chest pain 5
  Chest pain flowchart 5
Palpitations 12
  Palpitations flowchart 12
Breathlessness 19
  The breathless patient flowchart 19
Collapse/loss of consciousness (LOC) 33
  Collapsed patient flowchart 33
The patient with infection 43
  The patient with infection flowchart 43
Diabetes mellitus 53
Headache 56
  Headache flowchart 56
Poisoning 62
Severe allergic reaction 69
Thromboembolic problems 70
Environmental problems 72
Haematological problems 74
Psychiatry 76
Ophthalmology 84

CONTENTS

Chapter 2: SURGERY — 87
Abdominal pain — 88
   Abdominal pain flowchart — 88
Acute arterial occlusion — 105
Rectal bleeding — 107
Testicular pain — 111
   Testicular pain flowchart — 111
Gynaecology — 115
   Spontaneous miscarriage flowchart — 115
Orthopaedics — 119
   Joint problems flowchart — 119

Part B: INJURY — 127
Assault — 128
Major injury — 130
Burns — 132
Swallowed/inhaled foreign bodies — 134
Minor wound care — 136
Injury according to location — 146
   Canadian cervical spine rule flowchart — 156

Part C: INFANTS — 185
General information — 187
The unwell child — 188
Abdominal problems — 192
Breathlessness — 196
CNS problems and injury — 204
   Status epilepticus flowchart — 206
Injury — 207

INDEX — 217

Contact numbers — 235

Covers
   Glasgow coma scale — *inside front cover*
   Child's Glasgow coma scale
     (<4 years old) — *inside back cover*

PREFACE

It is an absolute pleasure to write this preface. Working in an Emergency Department is a fantastic cocktail of adrenaline and apprehension. There is no doubt that the Emergency Department is the most stimulating, rewarding, unpredictable and exciting environment in which you will ever work. Coupled with these emotions is undeniable anticipation. What on earth will come through the door next?!

Such apprehension is entirely healthy and normal! Every day we see large numbers of patients presenting with the entire spectrum of acute illness and injury. These are undifferentiated patients and usually, we are the first doctors to see them and determine whether or not their condition is serious or even life-threatening. For those patients who are obviously very ill or badly injured, we need a safe, simple, structured approach to their care, understanding which immediate interventions are indicated and when to call for more senior help. For the less seriously ill and injured patients, we must ensure that they also receive consistently high standards of care.

Fear not! Don't panic! – help is at hand!

In this excellent survival guide, the authors have produced a comprehensive but rapidly accessible collection of the key aspects of Emergency Medicine which will help you and the patient in your care.

It can be a jungle out there but this book will keep you safely out of tiger country!

John Heyworth MBChB FRCS FFAEM FIFEM

Consultant, Emergency Department
Southampton General Hospital

President of the British Association
for Accident and Emergency Medicine

INTRODUCTION

How to use this book

This book is designed to be used where you need it most – 'on the shop floor'. As such, it is not an exhaustive textbook that would weigh you down. Our aim is to have included those conditions that you may commonly see in any Emergency Department (ED). Sometimes the diagnosis is not clear and this book will help you come to a provisional diagnosis, using flowcharts of presenting symptoms.

The book is split into three sections, Illness, Injury and Infants; the symbols at the bottom of the page will help you find which section you are in.

If you think you know the diagnosis then go to the appropriate page where the important things to ask, to look for on examination, investigations to do and treatments are outlined. There are suggestions on whom to send home and whom to refer, as this can be one of the most difficult things to learn in the ED.

Knowing when to ask for help can also be hard. In the book if you see 'get help' at the top of the page be sure that your senior would want to know about the patient in front of you now, rather than after you have done all the listed investigations. Sometimes on 'what to look for' you may find something that means you should 'get help' immediately such as signs of shock. The sooner you call for help the sooner it will arrive!

By including drug dosages we do not want this book to take the place of the British National Formulary (BNF). You should know certain drug dosages and if you are not sure we advise checking with the BNF.

All ED's have their own policies and guidelines. Use this book to complement, not replace, those used in your department, there is space in the book to make a note of important information or specific guidelines.

INTRODUCTION

Finally, as you spend time in the ED you will learn quickly and become able to manage more and more illness or injuries. Use the book to remind yourself of the important points and think, 'how did we manage this last time?'

INTRODUCTION xi

Risks and difficulties of working in the emergency department
Practical risks

- Maintain patients' confidentiality at all times
- Assess all your patients holistically, eg a wrist fracture in the elderly may prevent mobility if their stick is normally held in that hand
- Most departments have regular attenders (often drug or alcohol abusers) – sooner or later they will come with a serious problem so always check them thoroughly
- 'Lucky' patients – significant history (eg hit by car) with little/no injury – get a second opinion

Communication difficulties

- The confused/intoxicated – history usually unreliable – ensure thorough examination (including head injury) and observations including capillary blood glucose
- Relatives and friends are often extremely valuable sources of vital information
- Patients may be frustrated, in pain or drunk – if faced by potential verbal or physical aggression
  - **Get help** – senior and /or security
  - Try to avoid reacting and attempt to explain
- Your written notes are vital – you may need to rely on them later – ensure they are clear and comprehensive

Looking after yourself

- Work with all the team – doctors, nurses, etc. – listen to all advice offered but don't forget the final decision, and the responsibility for it, is yours
- Take breaks – tired doctors make errors. If a mistake does occur don't be afraid to apologise
- Errors are often made by looking at the wrong X-ray – check it is the right patient and the right date
- If a patient wishes to make a complaint – **get help**

Give patients an option to return or advise them to see their GP if the problem doesn't settle or progress as planned

Giving pain relief

Assessing the need for analgesia

- There is enormous variability in pain perception and need for analgesia – assess each patient individually
- Use an objective assessment, eg a pain score
- Reassess after analgesia given

Prior to giving analgesia

- Don't forget simple techniques that may reduce analgesia requirement:
  - Reassurance and explanation
  - Splinting with a sling or temporary plaster
  - Dressing, eg for burns
  - Simple treatments, eg trephining a fingernail
- Consider all available methods of analgesia
  - Local anaesthetic (LA) blocks
  - Entonox
  - Combinations of analgesics, eg paracetamol + NSAID + opiate
- If unfamiliar with a particular LA technique or unsure of which type or route of analgesic to use – **Get help**

Giving analgesia

- Consider route of administration – oral analgesia has a variable effect and can take 15 min to start working
- Morphine is the standard drug for severe pain
- NSAIDs are useful in musculoskeletal and inflammatory conditions, but check contra-indications
- Make sure all your patients are discharged with adequate analgesia for their problem

A standard intravenous analgesia regime
- Make sure the patient is monitored
- Use 10 mg morphine made up to 10 ml with water – give slowly intravenously in 2 mg aliquots over a few minutes until pain has eased
- Don't forget an antiemetic in adults
- Don't be afraid to use more than 10 mg morphine if the pain isn't easing – be aware of side-effects, eg respiratory depression.

INTRODUCTION

Abbreviations

ABG	arterial blood gases
CVA	cerebrovascular accident
DVT	deep vein thrombosis
ECG	electrocardiogram
FBC	full blood count
GCS	Glasgow coma scale
ICU	intensive care unit
IV	intravenous
LFT	liver function test
NSAIDS	non-steroidal antiinflammatory drugs
PEFR	peak expiratory flow rate
PID	pelvic inflammatory disease
PMH	previous medical history
p.o.	per os (by mouth)
PR	per rectum
SaO_2	arterial oxygen saturation
SCA	sickle cell anaemia
SOB	shortness of breath
TIA	transient ischaemic attack
U&E's	urea and electrolytes

Table of normal haematological and biochemical values
Blood, serum and plasma

Haematology

Haemoglobin	12.5–14.5 g/dl
Mean corpuscular volume (MCV)	80–96 fl
Mean corpuscular haemoglobin (MCH)	28–32 pg
Mean corpuscular haemoglobin concentration (MCHC)	32–35 g/dl
White cell count (WCC)	$4–11 \times 10^9/l$
Differential WCC: Neutrophils	$1.5–7 \times 10^9/l$
Lymphocytes	$1.5–4 \times 10^9/l$
Eosinophils	$0.04–0.4 \times 10^9/l$
Platelet count	$150–400 \times 10^9/l$
Reticulocyte count	$50–100 \times 10^9/l$
Prothrombin time (PT)	12–17 s
Activated partial thromboplastin time (APTT)	24–38 s
Thrombin time (TT)	14–22 s
Fibrinogen	2–5 g/l
Fibrinogen degradation products (FDP)	<10 mcg/ml
International normalised ratio (INR)	<1.4
Erythrocyte sedimentation rate (ESR)	<12 mm/(1st) hour
Plasma viscosity	1.5–1.72 cP

Endocrinology

Fasting glucose	3.0–6.0 mmol/l
Thyroid stimulating hormone (TSH)	0.3–4.0 mU/l
Thyroxine (T4)	58–174 nmol/l
Free T4 (FT4)	10–24 pmol/l

Biochemistry

Sodium (Na⁺)	137–144 mmol/l
Potassium (K⁺)	3.5–4.9 mmol/l
Chloride	95–107 mmol/l
Urea	0–180 mcgmol/l
Creatinine	60–110 mcgmol/l
Calcium (Ca^{2+}), corrected	2.25–2.70 mmol/l
Phosphate	0.8–1.4 mmol/l
Creatine kinase (CK)	<120 U/l
Uric acid	0–0.43 mmol/l
Amylase	60–180 U/l
Alanine aminotransferase (ALT)	5–35 U/l
Aspartate aminotransferase (AST)	1–31 U/l
Alkaline phosphatase (ALP)	20–120 U/l
Lactate dehydrogenase (LDH)	10–250 U/l
Gamma-glutamyl transferase (GGT)	4–35 U/l (<50 U/l in men)
Bilirubin (total)	1–22 mcgmol/l
Total protein	61–76 g/l
Albumin	37–49 g/l
Cholesterol	<5.2 mmol/l
Triglyceride (fasting)	0.45–1.69 mmol/l

Blood gases

pH	7.36–7.44
PaO_2	11.3–12.6 kPa
$PaCO_2$	4.7–6.0 kPa
Bicarbonate	20–28 mmol/l

Therapeutic drug levels

Digoxin (≥ 6 h post-dose)	1–2 mcg/l
Lithium	0.4–1.0 mmol/l

Part A
ILLNESS

Chapter 1: MEDICAL — 3
Cardiac arrest — 4
Chest pain — 5
Palpitations — 12
Breathlessness — 19
Collapse/loss of consciousness (LOC) — 33
The patient with infection — 43
Diabetes mellitus — 53
Headache — 56
Poisoning — 62
Severe allergic reaction — 69
Thromboembolic problems — 70
Environmental problems — 72
Haematological problems — 74
Psychiatry — 76
Ophthalmology — 84

Chapter 2: SURGERY — 87
Abdominal pain — 88
Acute arterial occlusion — 105
Rectal bleeding — 107
Testicular pain — 111
Gynaecology — 115
Orthopaedics — 119

ILLNESS

Chapter 1
MEDICAL

ILLNESS

4 ILLNESS

Cardiac arrest
Cardiac arrest flowchart

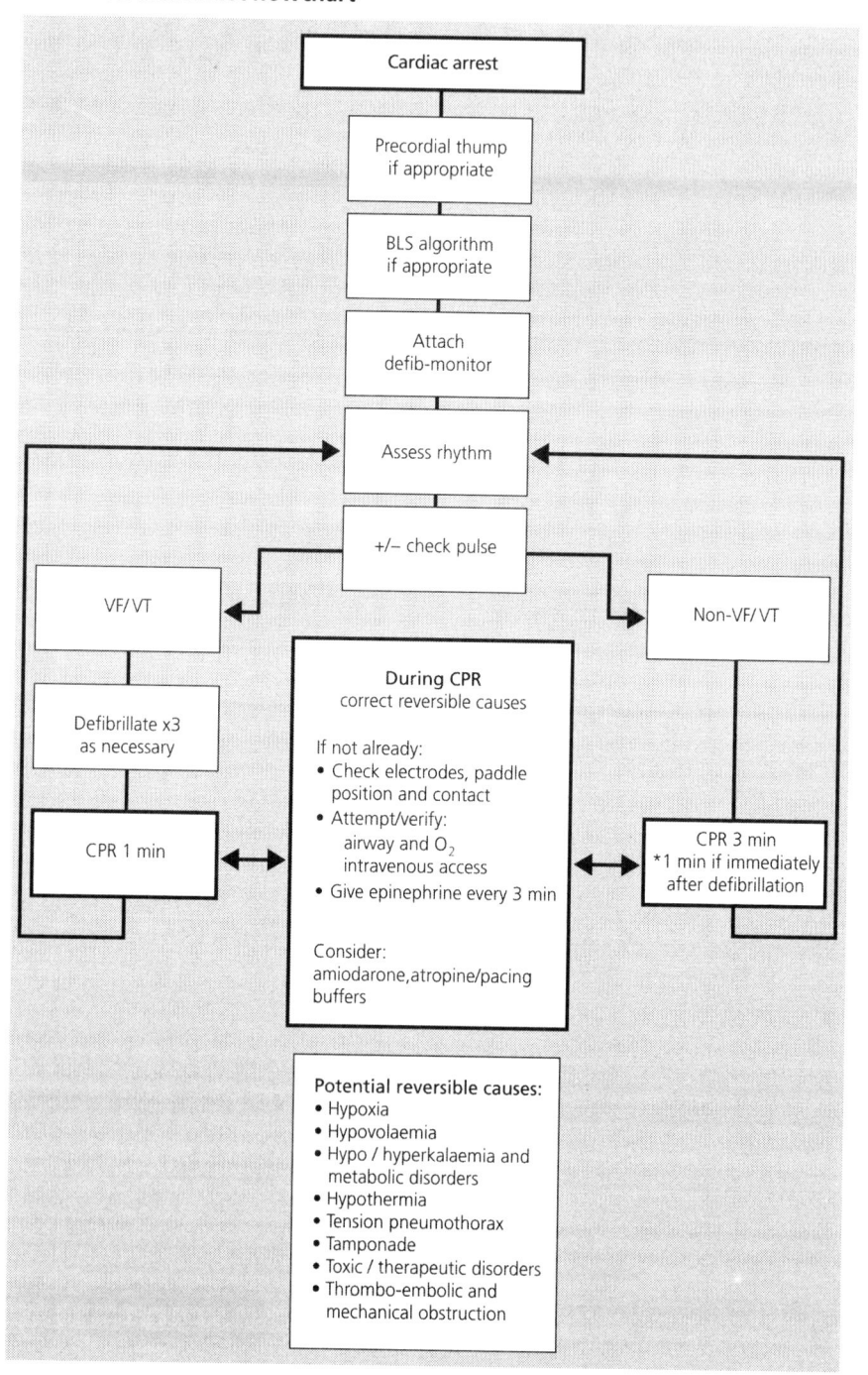

```
                    Cardiac arrest
                          │
                  Precordial thump
                   if appropriate
                          │
                   BLS algorithm
                   if appropriate
                          │
                      Attach
                   defib-monitor
                          │
                   Assess rhythm
                          │
                  +/− check pulse
                   ╱            ╲
              VF/VT            Non-VF/VT
                │                  │
         Defibrillate x3            │
          as necessary              │
                │                   │
            CPR 1 min   ⟷   CPR 3 min
                                *1 min if immediately
                                after defibrillation
```

During CPR
correct reversible causes

If not already:
- Check electrodes, paddle position and contact
- Attempt/verify: airway and O_2 intravenous access
- Give epinephrine every 3 min

Consider:
amiodarone, atropine/pacing buffers

Potential reversible causes:
- Hypoxia
- Hypovolaemia
- Hypo / hyperkalaemia and metabolic disorders
- Hypothermia
- Tension pneumothorax
- Tamponade
- Toxic / therapeutic disorders
- Thrombo-embolic and mechanical obstruction

MEDICAL 5

Chest pain

Please also refer to sections **Pulmonary embolism** (page 26–27) and **Spontaneous pneumothorax** (page 28–29)

Chest pain flowchart

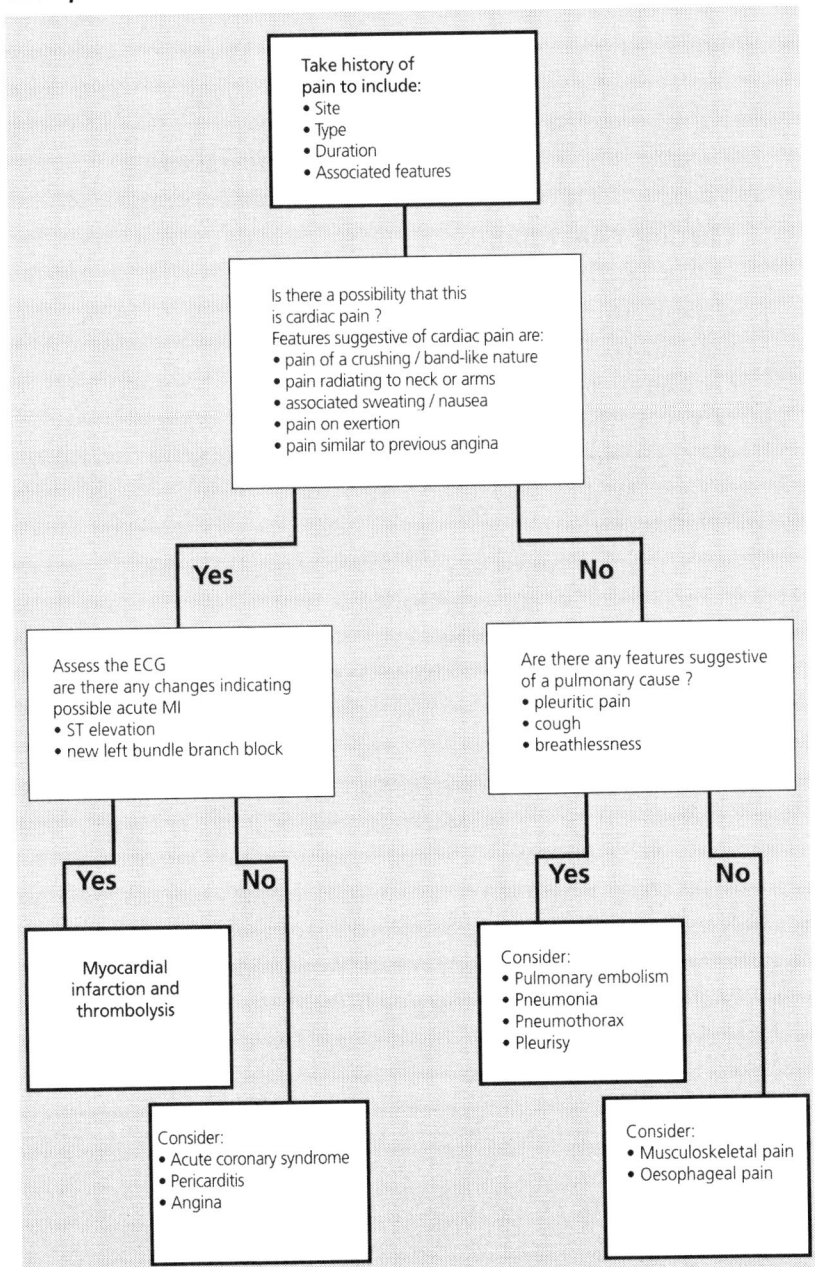

```
Take history of pain to include:
• Site
• Type
• Duration
• Associated features
        │
        ▼
Is there a possibility that this is cardiac pain?
Features suggestive of cardiac pain are:
• pain of a crushing / band-like nature
• pain radiating to neck or arms
• associated sweating / nausea
• pain on exertion
• pain similar to previous angina
```

Yes → Assess the ECG are there any changes indicating possible acute MI
- ST elevation
- new left bundle branch block

  - **Yes →** Myocardial infarction and thrombolysis
  - **No →** Consider:
    - Acute coronary syndrome
    - Pericarditis
    - Angina

No → Are there any features suggestive of a pulmonary cause?
- pleuritic pain
- cough
- breathlessness

  - **Yes →** Consider:
    - Pulmonary embolism
    - Pneumonia
    - Pneumothorax
    - Pleurisy
  - **No →** Consider:
    - Musculoskeletal pain
    - Oesophageal pain

Illness

Acute coronary syndromes

These include unstable angina and non-Q-wave infarcts. Consider if this is a myocardial infarction (see page 8–9)

What to ask

- For how long have they had the pain
- Does it sound cardiac in nature
- What were they doing when it started

Cardiac chest pain

- Crushing band-like pain around chest
- Radiation to neck, jaw or arm

Associated factors:
- Pain on exertion
- Previous ischaemic heart disease

What to look for

- Hypotension
- Crackles in lung bases
- Arrhythmias
- Associated features – sweating, clammy

Investigations

- FBC, U&E's, glucose, cardiac enzymes and cholesterol
- ECG showing ST depression or T wave inversion; may show no initial changes so repeat if pain changes or persists
- Chest X-ray

Cardiac enzymes used in my department are:

MEDICAL

Management

- 100% oxygen
- Cardiac monitoring
- 300 mg aspirin and 300 mg clopidrogrel unless true allergy
- Titrate IV morphine/diamorphine for analgesia and give antiemetic
- Consider low-molecular-weight heparins

Who needs referral

- Refer if need IV morphine/diamorphine
- Pain came on at rest
- Increasing episodes of angina
- Those who have had a simple anginal episode less than 10 minutes duration may be discharged if they are pain free and have a GP or imminent physician follow-up

ILLNESS

Myocardial infarction (MI)

Take the history at the same time as initiating treatments and remember 'time is myocardium'

What to ask

- When did the pain start
- Does it sound cardiac in nature
- Previous MI especially if thrombolytics been given before

Cardiac chest pain

- Crushing band-like pain around chest
- Radiation to neck, jaw or arm

Associated factors:
- Pain on exertion
- Previous ischaemic heart disease

What to look for

If signs of shock, tachycardia, prolonged capillary refill or hypotensive – **Get help**

- Sweating, clammy and in pain
- Crackles in lung bases

Investigations

- FBC, U&E's, glucose, cardiac enzymes and cholesterol
- ECG is diagnostic if ST segment elevation >1 mm in two adjacent limb leads or >2 mm in two or more adjacent chest leads or new left bundle branch block (LBBB)
- Chest X-ray

MEDICAL

Management

- **Get help**
- 100% oxygen
- Cardiac monitoring
- 300 mg aspirin and 300 mg clopidrogrel unless true allergy
- Titrate IV morphine/diamorphine for analgesia and give antiemetic
- Thrombolysis after exclusion of contraindications and informed consent by patient. Check your department's protocol

Who needs referral

- Refer all to on-call physicians

My department's thrombolysis protocol:

ILLNESS

Pericarditis

Inflammation of the pericardial sac around the heart

What to ask

- Nature of chest pain
- Recent flu-like illness or pyrexia
- Recent cardiac surgery or myocardial infarction
- Central chest pain, worse on sitting forward and stabbing in nature

What to look for

- Pericardial friction rub over the heart
- Engorged neck veins, hypotension and breathlessness suggesting cardiac tamponade – **Get help**

Investigations

- Concave, curving upwards, or saddle-shaped ST elevation across many leads on ECG
- FBC, U&E's, C-reactive protein
- Cardiac enlargement on chest X-ray

Management

- Titrate IV morphine/diamorphine for analgesia and give antiemetic

Who needs referral

- Refer all to on-call physicians

MEDICAL

Chest pain – diagnosis uncertain

The following must be done for **all** patients with chest pain:
- Thorough history including cardiac risk factors
- Examination including chest and abdomen
- Observations:
  - Pulse
  - Blood pressure
  - Oxygen saturation
  - Capillary blood glucose
- Two ECGs 30 min apart if there is **any** possibility of cardiac pain

Commonly misused diagnoses

- 'Musculoskeletal chest pain' – in the absence of a definite history of injury this is rare
- 'Costochondritis' – be aware that pressure on the chest reproducing pain may be found in ischaemic cardiac pain and pulmonary embolism
- 'Indigestion' – unusual as a cause of chest pain presenting to an Emergency Department. Beware – antacids may relieve cardiac pain, and nausea and vomiting often accompany chest pain
- 'Non-cardiac chest pain' – just because the ECG and enzymes are normal does not exclude cardiac pain. One-third of initial ECGs are normal in acute MI and cardiac enzymes may take 12 h to become abnormal

ECG interpretation

- Two ECGs are usually easier to interpret than one
- Changes on the second compared to the first should prompt admission
- Use old ECGs to assess new changes
- If you aren't sure get another opinion
- The computer diagnosis produced by many machines should be treated with the same authority as a medical student

ILLNESS

Palpitations

Palpitations flowchart

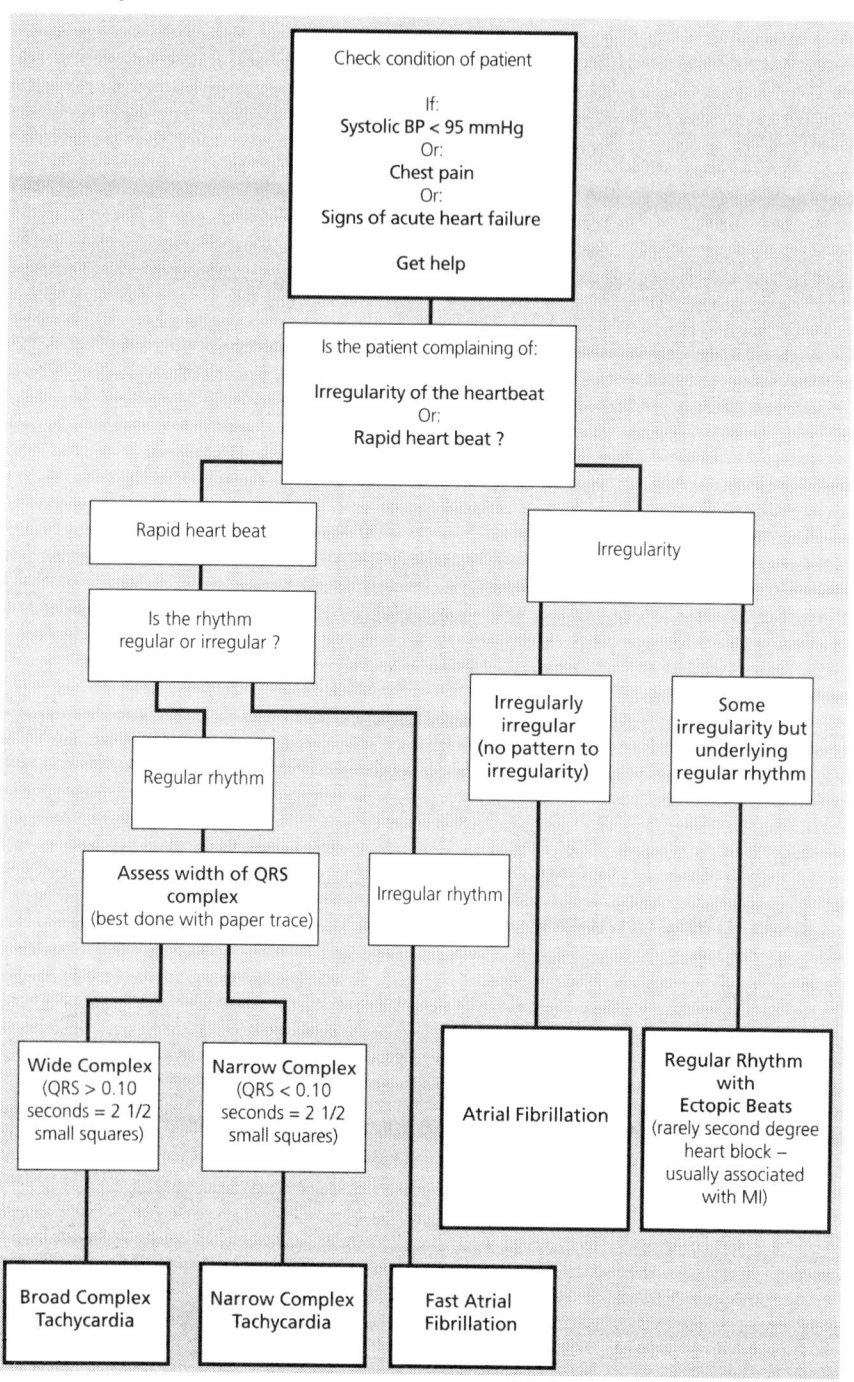

Check condition of patient

If:
Systolic BP < 95 mmHg
Or:
Chest pain
Or:
Signs of acute heart failure

Get help

↓

Is the patient complaining of:

Irregularity of the heartbeat
Or:
Rapid heart beat?

- **Rapid heart beat**
  - Is the rhythm regular or irregular?
    - **Regular rhythm**
      - Assess width of QRS complex (best done with paper trace)
        - **Wide Complex** (QRS > 0.10 seconds = 2 1/2 small squares) → **Broad Complex Tachycardia**
        - **Narrow Complex** (QRS < 0.10 seconds = 2 1/2 small squares) → **Narrow Complex Tachycardia**
    - **Irregular rhythm** → **Fast Atrial Fibrillation**

- **Irregularity**
  - **Irregularly irregular** (no pattern to irregularity) → **Atrial Fibrillation**
  - **Some irregularity but underlying regular rhythm** → **Regular Rhythm with Ectopic Beats** (rarely second degree heart block – usually associated with MI)

MEDICAL

Broad complex tachycardia

What to look for on the ECG

- Fast rate – usually >120 beats per minute
- Regular rhythm
- Broad complexes – QRS duration >0.10 seconds, ie greater than $2\frac{1}{2}$ small squares

For all patients with a broad complex tachycardia – Get help

Before help arrives check if the patient has any adverse signs:
- Systolic BP < 95 mmHg
- Chest pain
- Signs of acute heart failure – eg pulmonary oedema, raised jugular venous pressure
- Rate 150 beats per minute or more

If **any** of these are present then the patient will need electrical cardioversion as soon as possible

If **no** adverse signs are present then drug treatment is required. This will depend on whether the rhythm is:
- Ventricular tachycardia (VT) or
- Supraventricular tachycardia (SVT) with aberrant conduction (bundle branch block)
- Discuss this decision with a senior or a physician

Investigations

- FBC, U&E's, glucose, cardiac enzymes (according to local policy)
- Chest X-ray

Management

- All patient should receive high-flow oxygen
- Treatment – for both cardioversion and drug treatment find out your departmental policy
- All patients should be referred to a physician

ILLNESS

Narrow complex tachycardia

What to look for on the ECG

- Fast rate – usually >150 beats per minute
- Regular rhythm – an irregular rhythm normally means fast atrial fibrillation (see page 16–17)
- Narrow complexes QRS duration ≤0.10 seconds, ie 2½ small squares or less
- Signs of ischaemia – ST depression or T inversion

What to ask

- Previous episodes

What to look for

- Adverse signs
  - Systolic BP < 95 mmHg
  - Chest pain
  - Signs of acute heart failure, eg pulmonary oedema, raised jugular venous pressure
  - Rate 200 beats per minute or more
  - Reduced conscious level

If **any** of these are present then **Get help**

Management

- If **no** adverse signs are present then consider
  - Vagal manoeuvres, eg valsalva manoeuvre – blowing in the end of a 20-ml syringe trying to push the plunger out works well
  - Carotid sinus massage – avoid if carotid bruit
  - Adenosine (see Box)

MEDICAL

Using adenosine

- Get help if you haven't used adenosine before
- If patient is asthmatic or taking dipyridamole – discuss with senior/physician
- Inject into ante-cubital fossa vein with rapid flush of 20 ml saline
- Start with 6 mg dose; if no response give 12 mg then further 12 mg
- Warn the patient they will feel terrible for a few seconds
- Make sure you are recording a rhythm trace: there should be a pause and then hopefully sinus rhythm
- If adenosine isn't successful **Get help**

Admit patients if

- Adenosine doesn't work
- Ischaemic changes on the ECG at any time
- Elderly
- Recurrent recent episodes

ILLNESS

Atrial fibrillation (AF)

What to look for on the ECG

- Irregularly irregular rhythm
- Complexes usually narrow
- Rate
- Signs of ischaemia – ST depression or T inversion

> **Fast AF (rate >100 beats per minute) can:**
> - be a primary arrhythmia in someone who is normally in sinus rhythm **or**
> - occur as a secondary response to pain/shock/fever, etc. in someone with known AF

What to ask

- Is the atrial fibrillation new or previously known
  If new onset:
  - Try to ascertain when first noticed
  If known AF:
  - is rate normally controlled and what with
- Neurological symptoms – consider an embolic event

What to look for

- Signs of shock – prolonged capillary return, tachycardia, hypotension, altered mental state – **Get help**
- Signs of acute heart failure, eg crackles in lungs

Investigations

- FBC, U&E's, glucose
- Thyroid function tests – if new-onset AF
- Chest X-ray

MEDICAL

Management

- If any signs of shock or acute heart failure – **Get help**
- If the patient is in fast AF consider a possible underlying secondary cause and treat appropriately, eg give analgesia/treat fever
- If new-onset AF and the patient is stable refer to a physician

ILLNESS

Palpitations – diagnosis uncertain

If the ECG is normal

- Keep the patient on a monitor for 30-60 min and ask them to let you know if they feel the palpitations

If still normal

- Reassure and ask to return if further prolonged episode
- Stress and anxiety may cause an increased frequency of ectopics or make them more noticeable – reassure the patient

If the ECG shows ectopic beats

- Decide if they are supraventricular or ventricular
- They are ventricular if:
  - the complex is more than $2\frac{1}{2}$ small squares wide
  - looks different from the 'normal' complexes

Ventricular ectopics are worrying if they

- Are frequent (more ectopics than normal complexes)
- Are multifocal (they have different shapes)
- Occur in runs
  - 2 in a row   = a couplet
  - 3 in a row   = a salvo
  - 4 or more in a row = broad complex tachycardia
- Occur close to the preceding complex – if the ectopic hits the preceding T wave (R on T phenomenon) it can trigger ventricular fibrillation or tachycardia

Who to admit

- Always refer patients with worrying ectopics
- If occasional ventricular ectopics are seen with no worrying features then reassure the patient
- In general supraventricular ectopics are harmless and reassurance is all that is needed

MEDICAL 19

Breathlessness
The breathless patient flowchart

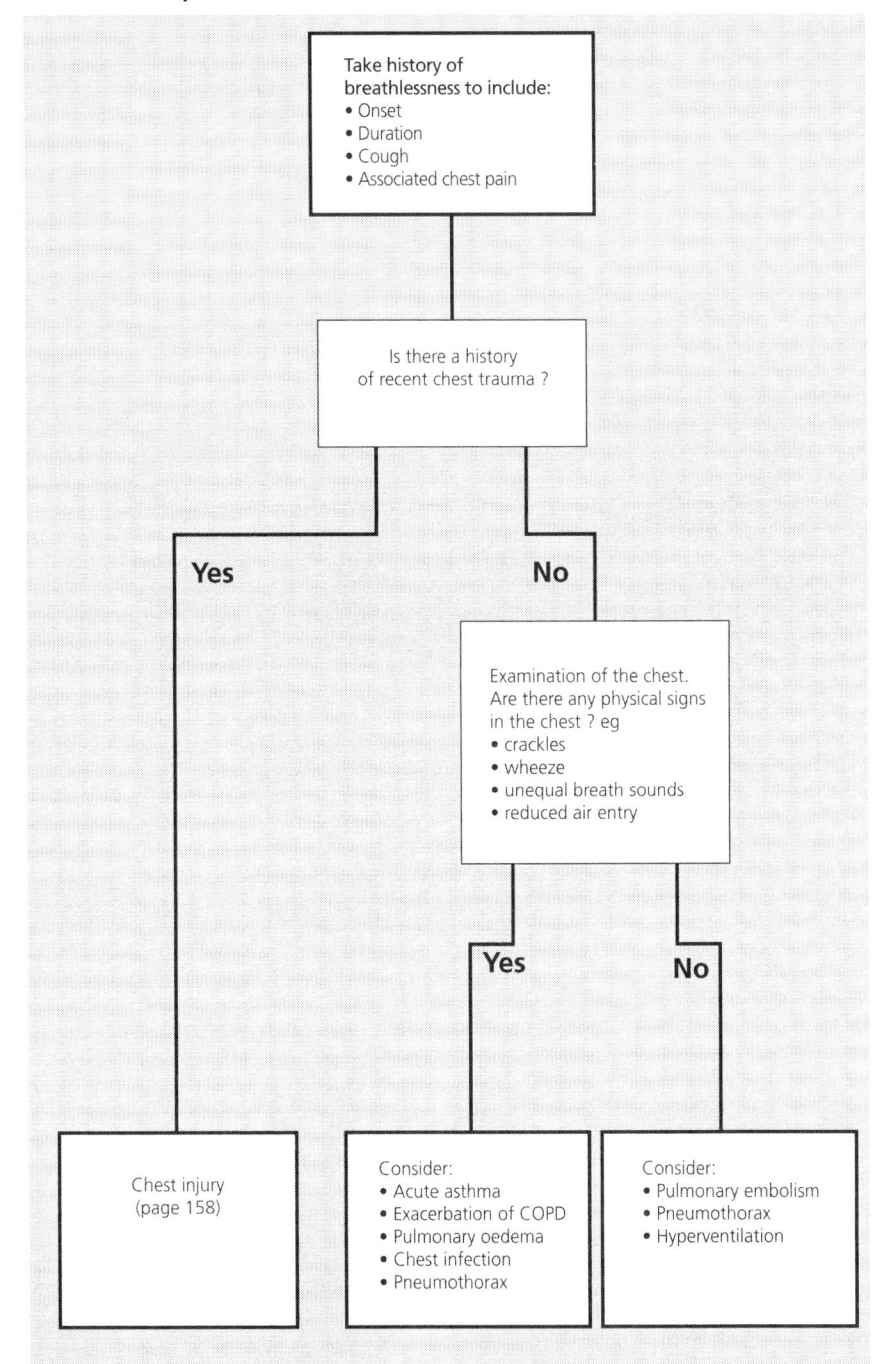

```
┌─────────────────────────────┐
│ Take history of             │
│ breathlessness to include:  │
│  • Onset                    │
│  • Duration                 │
│  • Cough                    │
│  • Associated chest pain    │
└─────────────────────────────┘
              │
┌─────────────────────────────┐
│ Is there a history          │
│ of recent chest trauma ?    │
└─────────────────────────────┘
       │                │
      Yes              No
       │                │
       │    ┌─────────────────────────────┐
       │    │ Examination of the chest.   │
       │    │ Are there any physical signs│
       │    │ in the chest ? eg           │
       │    │  • crackles                 │
       │    │  • wheeze                   │
       │    │  • unequal breath sounds    │
       │    │  • reduced air entry        │
       │    └─────────────────────────────┘
       │              │           │
       │             Yes         No
       │              │           │
┌──────────────┐ ┌─────────────────────┐ ┌──────────────────────┐
│ Chest injury │ │ Consider:           │ │ Consider:            │
│ (page 158)   │ │ • Acute asthma      │ │ • Pulmonary embolism │
│              │ │ • Exacerbation of   │ │ • Pneumothorax       │
│              │ │   COPD              │ │ • Hyperventilation   │
│              │ │ • Pulmonary oedema  │ │                      │
│              │ │ • Chest infection   │ │                      │
│              │ │ • Pneumothorax      │ │                      │
└──────────────┘ └─────────────────────┘ └──────────────────────┘
```

ILLNESS

Asthma

What to ask

- Onset
- Chest tightness, wheeze, cough, shortness of breath
- Previous hospital/ ICU admissions
- Nocturnal symptoms
- Increase in frequency of symptoms
- Recent steroids
- Recent infection

What to look for

	Moderate	Severe	Life-threatening
Peak expiratory flow rate (PEFR)	>50%	<50%	<33%
Respiratory rate (breaths per minute)	<25	>25	Silent chest
Pulse (beats per minute)	<110	>110	Bradycardia
Ability to speak	Full sentences	Unable to complete full sentences	Confusion, exhaustion, coma

Immediate treatment

- Keep calm!
- PEFR if possible
- High-flow oxygen
- Nebuliser: 5 mg salbutamol and 500 mcg atrovent
- Prednisolone 40 mg p.o. or 200 mg IV hydrocortisone
- Repeat salbutamol nebuliser if needed every 15 min

If your patient deteriorates or shows no signs of improvement **Get help** You may need to consider IV aminophylline or IV salbutamol and magnesium.

MEDICAL

Investigations

- ABG
- Chest X-ray: rule out a pneumothorax, infection
- FBC, U&E's, glucose
- Keep reassessing and reassuring your patient

ABG – worrying results
- Normal, rising, high CO_2
- Severe hypoxia PaO_2<8 kPa on high-flow O_2

Get help

Who to admit

- All life threatening and severe asthmatics should be admitted.
- All other patients should be discussed with a senior or on-call physician
- If sending patient home ensure they have GP follow-up

- Severity of wheeze is a poor guide to the severity of asthma
- Nebulisers should be driven by oxygen not air
- Underestimation of severity by patient/ doctor kills!

ILLNESS

Chest infection

What to ask

- Cough, pyrexia, rigors, shortness of breath, sputum, haemoptysis
- Presence and character of pain
- PMH: asthma, chronic obstructive pulmonary disease (COPD), HIV, cancer
- Recent foreign travel
- Smoker

What to look for

- Pyrexia
- Dyspnoea, tachycardia
- Confusion, particularly in the elderly
- Crackles, bronchial breathing, decreased breath sounds

CURB
- **C**onfusion, new or GCS < 8
- **U**rea > 7mmol/l
- **R**espiratory rate > 30/min
- **B**lood pressure low systolic < 90 mmHg and /or diastolic < 60 mmHg

Get help if any of the above are present

Investigations

- FBC, U&E's, glucose, blood cultures
- Sputum sample, mid-stream urine sample
- ABG if arterial oxygen saturation (SaO_2) < 92% on room air
- Chest X-ray: diffuse shadowing, pleural effusion, lobar consolidation

MEDICAL

Management

Use the British Thoracic Society (BTS) adverse prognostic features (CURB) and clinical judgement:
- High-flow oxygen
- Analgesia, paracetamol and/or NSAID
- Antibiotics, p.o. or IV, refer to your hospital policy
- Consider nebulisers for bronchospasm

My department's antibiotic policy for chest infection:

Who to admit

- Discharge home with GP follow-up and antibiotics if no adverse prognostic features or young with a single lobe affected
- Refer to physicians if PMH of cancer or chronic lung disease
- Refer if one or more adverse prognostic features

ILLNESS

ILLNESS

Chronic obstructive pulmonary disease (COPD)

What to ask

- Recent course of disease
- Increasing breathlessness, wheeze
- Increase in amount or change in colour of purulent sputum
- Decrease in exercise tolerance
- Home oxygen, nebulisers
- Previous admissions to ICU
- PMH

What to look for

- Tachypnoea
- Use of accessory muscles
- Cyanosis
- Wheeze, crepitations
- Decreased air entry
- Confusion, agitation – **Get help**

Investigations

- Oxygen saturation and temperature
- ABG
- FBC, U&E's, glucose, blood and sputum cultures
- Chest X-ray
- Old notes

ABG

Look at:
- pH is the best guide to a patient's exacerbation
- Patients die more quickly from hypoxia than hypercarbia!

MEDICAL

Management

- Sit upright
- High-flow oxygen initially; aim for SaO_2 > 92%
- 5 mg salbutamol and 500 mcg atrovent nebuliser
- Consider steroids, 40 mg prednisolone p.o. **or** 200 mg IV hydrocortisone
- If there is no improvement **Get help** – as you may need to consider IV salbutamol or aminophylline
- Consider antibiotics and non-invasive ventilation according to departmental policy

Who to admit

- Patients with a significant infection
- Patients who are unable to cope at home
- Patients with a deteriorating condition

My department's antibiotic policy for COPD:

ILLNESS

Pulmonary embolus (PE)

What to ask

- Breathlessness
- Pleuritic chest pain, worse on deep inspiration
- Haemoptysis
- Symptoms of DVT
- Risk factors:
  - malignancy
  - immobility
  - travel
  - oral contraceptives
  - hormone replacement therapy
  - pregnancy
  - previous thromboembolic disease

What to look for

- Tachypnoea/tachycardia
- Pleural rub
- Signs of shock: prolonged capillary refill, tachycardia, hypotension – **Get help**

Investigations

- FBC, U&E's, glucose, D-dimer
- ABG: hypoxia or hypercarbia
- Chest X-ray: help exclude other causes
- ECG: most commonly sinus tachycardia or evidence of right heart strain, eg right bundle branch block, S1Q3T3 (S wave in lead 1, Q wave lead 3, T wave inversion lead 3), atrial fibrillation

Management

- High-flow oxygen
- Titrate IV morphine for analgesia and give antiemetic
- Low molecular weight heparin, according to your hospital policy

MEDICAL

Who to admit

- You must work within your hospital policy; you need to know how sensitive and specific your lab D-dimer test is
- All patients with a high clinical probability need to be referred to the physicians
- Discuss intermediate probability cases with the physician

- All patients should be assessed on clinical probability
- D-dimer is to be considered following clinical probability; it should not be done on patients with high clinical probability
- A negative D-dimer excludes PE in patients with low/intermediate clinical probability

Spontaneous pneumothorax

Ask yourself, 'does this patient have a tension pneumothorax?' If yes, **Treat immediately!**

Signs of tension pneumothorax
- Tachycardic/tachypnoeic
- Tracheal diversion
- Hyper-resonance
- No breath sounds
- Collapse, in extremesis

Immediate thoracocentesis! – Get help

What to ask

- History of chest trauma
- Chronic lung disease
- Recent decrease in exercise tolerance
- Shortness of breath ?Sudden onset
- Chest pain – usually pleuritic pain
- Previous history of pneumothorax

Management

- High-flow oxygen
- Oxygen saturation and blood pressure
- Chest X-ray, **except in tension**

	Small collapse	Moderate/complete collapse
Signs/ symptoms	Often no symptoms	↓ Expansion ↓ Breath Sounds ↑ Resonance Dyspnoea
Treatment	If chronic lung disease, aspirate	Aspiration. If unsuccessful consider a chest drain **Get help**
Referral	Follow-up in 1/52 No diving No air travel	If remains expanded, discharge If chest drain needed, refer to physicians

MEDICAL

Procedures

Make sure you do the right thing to the right side!
- Needle thoracocentesis: insert a large bore cannula into the 2nd intercostal space at mid-clavicular line
- Chest drain insertion: 5th intercostal space, anterior to mid-axillary line

Left ventricular failure (pulmonary oedema)

What to ask

- Chest pain
- Exertional dyspnoea
- Orthopnoea/paroxysmal nocturnal dyspnoea
- Previous history MI, LVF
- Missed diuretics

What to look for

- Signs of shock: clammy/sweaty/anxious
- Dyspnoea/difficulty talking
- Tachycardic/tachypnoeic
- Pink frothy sputum
- Crackles or wheeze
- Heart murmurs, S3 gallop rhythm
- Signs of exhaustion/reduced level of consciousness – **Get help**

Investigations

- FBC, U/E's, glucose, cardiac enzymes and cholesterol
- ABG: look for hypoxia and/or hypercapnia
- Chest X-ray: upper lobe diversion/fluffy shadowing/bat's wings appearance/cardiomegaly/pleural effusion
- ECG: may show ischaemia, infarction, arrhythmia

Management

- **Keep calm**
- High flow oxygen
- Frusemide 50 mg IV
- Diamorphine up to 5 mg given slowly in 1 mg aliquots depending on patient's level of consciousness. Also give an antiemetic (not cyclizine)
- GTN spray and/or buccal or IV infusion according to your department's policy, if BP > 85 mmHg

MEDICAL

GTN infusion

50 mg in 50 ml 0.9% saline

Start at 2 mg/h and adjust according to clinical condition and blood pressure

Who needs referral

Refer all patients to the on-call physician

Breathlessness – diagnosis uncertain

What must be done for all patients with breathlessness:

- Thorough history
- Examination including cardiac and neurological
- Observations
  - Pulse
  - Blood pressure
  - Respiratory rate
  - Oxygen saturation
- ABG if the oxygen saturation is low or the diagnosis is in doubt – use local anaesthetic prior to taking the sample unless urgent

---

ABG interpretation

- Check pH – is there an acidosis or an alkalosis?
- Assess PCO_2 – an indication of the respiratory system
- Assess base excess – an indication of the metabolic system
- Interpret the PO_2 – dependent on the inspired percentage of oxygen

As an approximation in a patient with healthy lungs:
PO_2 in kPa = inspired oxygen percentage – 9 kPa

Non-pulmonary causes of breathlessness:

- Cardiac – eg arrhythmias (palpitations), myocardial infarction, left ventricular failure
- Neurological/muscular – neurological or muscular problems causing diaphragmatic weakness, eg Guillain-Barré syndrome, myasthenia gravis
- Metabolic – tachypnoea caused by metabolic acidosis, eg diabetic ketoacidosis, salicylate poisoning
- Hyperventilation/anxiety – **always** a diagnosis of exclusion. Be absolutely sure before you start treating a breathless patient by putting a paper bag over their face

MEDICAL

Collapse – loss of consciousness

Please also refer to the section on Subarachnoid haemorrhage (see page 57).

Collapsed patient flowchart

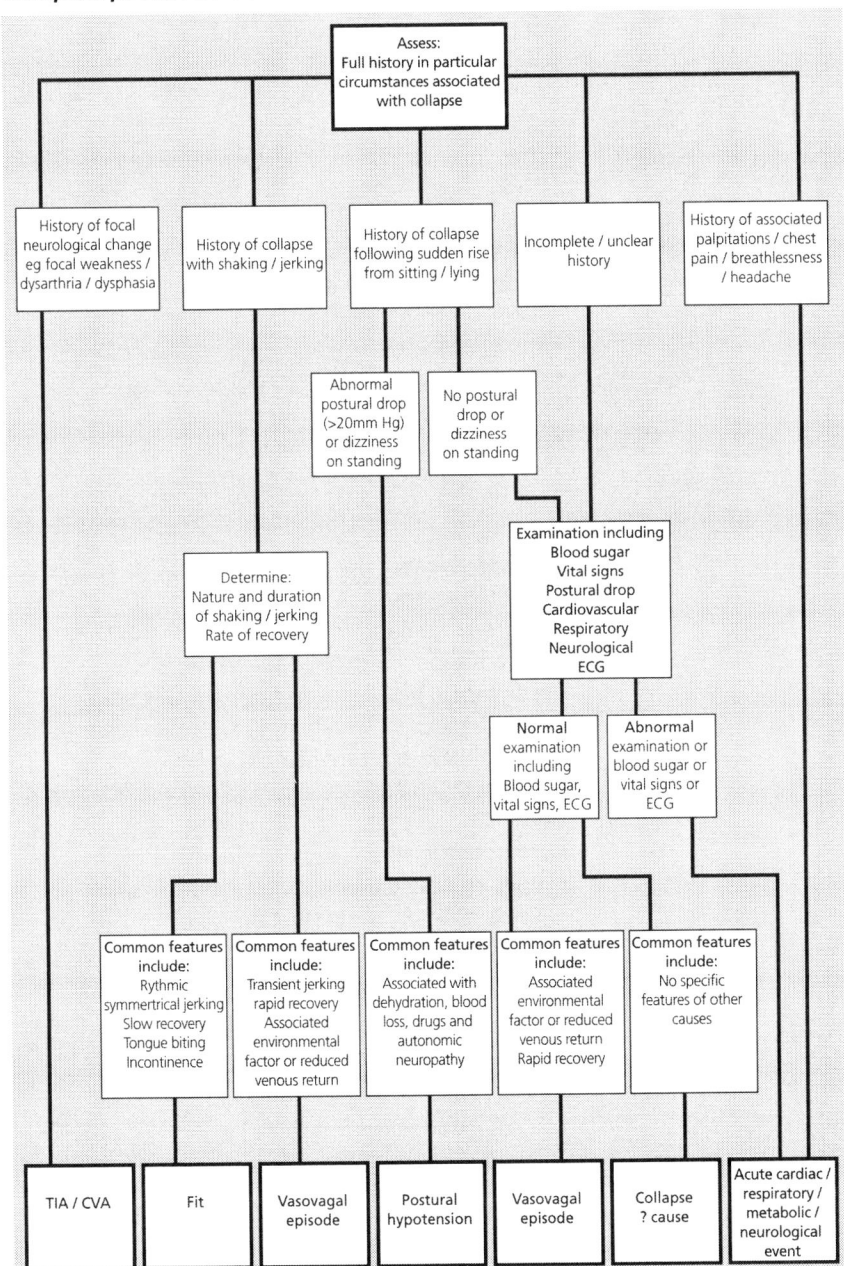

Assess: Full history in particular circumstances associated with collapse

Branches from assessment:

- **History of focal neurological change** eg focal weakness / dysarthria / dysphasia
- **History of collapse with shaking / jerking**
- **History of collapse following sudden rise from sitting / lying**
  - Abnormal postural drop (>20mm Hg) or dizziness on standing
  - No postural drop or dizziness on standing
- **Incomplete / unclear history**
- **History of associated palpitations / chest pain / breathlessness / headache**

Determine: Nature and duration of shaking / jerking, Rate of recovery

Examination including: Blood sugar, Vital signs, Postural drop, Cardiovascular, Respiratory, Neurological, ECG

- Normal examination including Blood sugar, vital signs, ECG
- Abnormal examination or blood sugar or vital signs or ECG

Common features include:

Column	Features	Outcome
1	Rythmic symmertrical jerking, Slow recovery, Tongue biting, Incontinence	—
2	Transient jerking rapid recovery, Associated environmental factor or reduced venous return	—
3	Associated with dehydration, blood loss, drugs and autonomic neuropathy	—
4	Associated environmental factor or reduced venous return, Rapid recovery	—
5	No specific features of other causes	—

Outcomes:
- TIA / CVA
- Fit
- Vasovagal episode
- Postural hypotension
- Vasovagal episode
- Collapse ? cause
- Acute cardiac / respiratory / metabolic / neurological event

ILLNESS

The unconscious patient

If asked to see an unconscious patient

- **Get help**
- Check ABC, give high-flow oxygen and, if no history of trauma, put in recovery position

What to ask

- There may be little or no history; get further details from:
  - Paramedics
  - Relatives
  - Hospital notes of previous attendances
  - GP
- Known diabetes
- Known drug or alcohol abuse
- Known epilepsy
- History of recent head injury

What to look for

- Responsiveness – use either
  - AVPU (*see* Box)
  - Glasgow coma scale (GCS; *see* inside front cover)
- Signs of shock – prolonged capillary refill, tachycardia, hypotension; if present **Get help**
- Hypoglycaemia – sweating, tachycardia, pallor
- Signs of new or recent head injury
- Continuing fit/epilepsy, eg minor jerking/flickering of eyelids
- Signs of drug abuse, eg needle marks
- Pupils – pinpoint usually indicates either opiate overdose or brainstem stroke

MEDICAL

> **The AVPU scale**
> A **A**lert
> V Responds to **v**oice
> P Responds to **p**ain
> U **U**nconscious
> P or U correspond to a GCS of 8 or less and the airway is at risk

Investigations

- Capillary blood glucose – if low **treat immediately**
- FBC, U&E's, glucose and further investigations depending on possible cause
- ECG
- Chest X-ray

Management

- Hypoglycaemia – 50–100 ml of 20% dextrose IV **or** 1 mg of glucagon IM (may not work in alcoholics)
- Opiate overdose – naloxone 800 mcg IV – repeat until no further improvement; if addict also give naloxone 800 mcg IM as patients often leave after rousing

Stroke (cerebrovascular accident, CVA) and transient ischaemic attack (TIA)

What to ask

- Focal neurological symptoms
- Headache
- Drug history – anticoagulants
- Risk factors

Risk factors for stroke/TIA

- Hypertension
- Atrial fibrillation
- Diabetes
- Ischaemic heart disease
- Smoking
- High cholesterol
- Oral contraceptive pill

What to look for

- Focal neurological signs – including cerebellar function, ie ataxia/vertigo/nystagmus
- Reduced level of consciousness – **Get help**
- Carotid bruit
- Ensure no other cause for neurological deficit:
  - Head injury
  - Infection, eg meningitis
  - Subarachnoid haemorrhage
  - Bell's palsy

Investigations

- Capillary blood glucose measurement – hypoglycaemia can present with a focal neurological deficit
- FBC, U&E's, glucose, lipid profile
- ECG
- Chest X-ray

MEDICAL

Management

If residual neurological signs or symptoms arrange admission:

Before admitting to the ward / stroke unit
- Give oxygen
- Start IV fluids
- Keep nil by mouth or arrange for a swallowing assessment

If neurological symptoms have settled and there are **no** neurological signs:

The patient can be discharged with GP follow-up only if:
- They are able to stand/walk as normal AND
- The blood pressure is normal AND
- All investigations are normal AND
- You have identified and given advice on any risk factors AND
- The patient is already on aspirin – if not start low-dose aspirin (75 mg) ensuring no contraindications

Vasovagal syncope (faint)

What to ask

- Circumstances of collapse:
  - Environment, eg hot stuffy room, sudden shock
  - Situation, eg micturition/prolonged standing
  - Eating – recent large meal/not eaten + exertion
- Careful history of collapse including presence of:
  - Prodrome, ie nausea, visual/aural disturbance
  - Chest pain (see page 5)
  - Palpitations (see page 12)
  - Breathlessness (see page 19)
  - Shaking/jerking during collapse
  - Recovery time
- Past history – previous episodes
- Drug history – any new medication or nitrate induced

What to look for

- If reduced level of consciousness – **Get help**
- Tongue biting
- Incontinence
- Rate and regularity of pulse
- Postural hypotension or dizziness on standing
- Consider occult GI bleeding (see page 109)

Investigations

- Capillary blood glucose measurement
- ECG
- FBC, U&E's, glucose, etc. – if not clearly a simple faint

Management

- Differentiate between a simple faint and a collapse

  Patients with simple faints
  - Usually have a precipitating cause and prodromal symptoms
  - Do not have chest pain/dyspnoea/palpitations

MEDICAL

- May transiently jerk/twitch
- Rarely are incontinent/bite their tongues
- Make a rapid recovery
- Examination and investigations are all normal

Patients with simple faints can be discharged home with advice

---

Collapsed patients:
- All other patients should be considered for admission and investigation – discuss with a senior or a physician

Fit/epilepsy

What to ask

If known to have epilepsy:
- Normal medication
- Normal frequency of fits and recent seizure pattern
- If recent change in seizure pattern – any current illness or other potential cause of the change

If this is a first fit:
- Circumstances and nature of fit in detail
- Symptoms of possible causes, eg:
  - Meningitis or other intracranial pathology
  - Head injury
  - Drug / alcohol ingestion or withdrawal

If the patient is still fitting
- **Get help**
- Check ABC, give high-flow oxygen and put in recovery position
- Get IV access – give lorazepam 0.1 mg/kg at 2 mg/min
- Check capillary blood glucose – if low give 50–100 ml 20% IV dextrose

If the fit persists beyond 5 min – get immediate help from a senior or a physician

---

What to look for

- If post-ictal – put in recovery position and give oxygen
- Full cardiovascular, respiratory and neurological examination for cause of fit or neurological deficit
- Injuries

Investigations

- Capillary blood glucose
- FBC, U&E's, blood glucose
- Blood cultures, ABG, ECG, chest X-ray, etc. if indicated

MEDICAL

Management

The patient can be discharged home if:
- They have made a full recovery
- There is a carer to watch them for the next few hours
- In a known epileptic there is no change in their normal seizure pattern and they have enough medication
- In a patient who has had a first fit and the examination and investigations are all normal. Advise the patient not to drive and to see their GP as soon as possible

All other patients should be discussed with a senior or a physician.

Collapse – diagnosis uncertain

Other causes of collapse

Cardiac syncope

Stokes Adams attack
- Usually associated with a cardiac arrhythmia
- Usually no warning and little/no symptoms
- Examination and ECG may be normal

Other cardiovascular disease
- Usually associated with exertion
- Causes can be:
  - Cardiac ischaemia and infarction
  - Aortic stenosis
  - Cardiomyopathy
- Examination and ECG usually abnormal

If a cardiac cause for syncope is found discuss with a senior or a physician

Postural hypotension (orthostatic hypotension)
- Collapse following rise from sitting/lying
- Measure postural drop (>20 mmHg is abnormal)
- Dizziness on standing is also significant

Often the cause of a collapse is not found in the Emergency department

It is safe to send home a patient following a collapse if:
- The collapse was short-lasting with a rapid recovery
- Examination and investigations are all normal
- The patient has someone to care for them at home
- The carer should be a healthy adult who is clear when to seek help

All other patients should be discussed with a senior or a physician.

MEDICAL 43

The patient with infection
The patient with infection flowchart

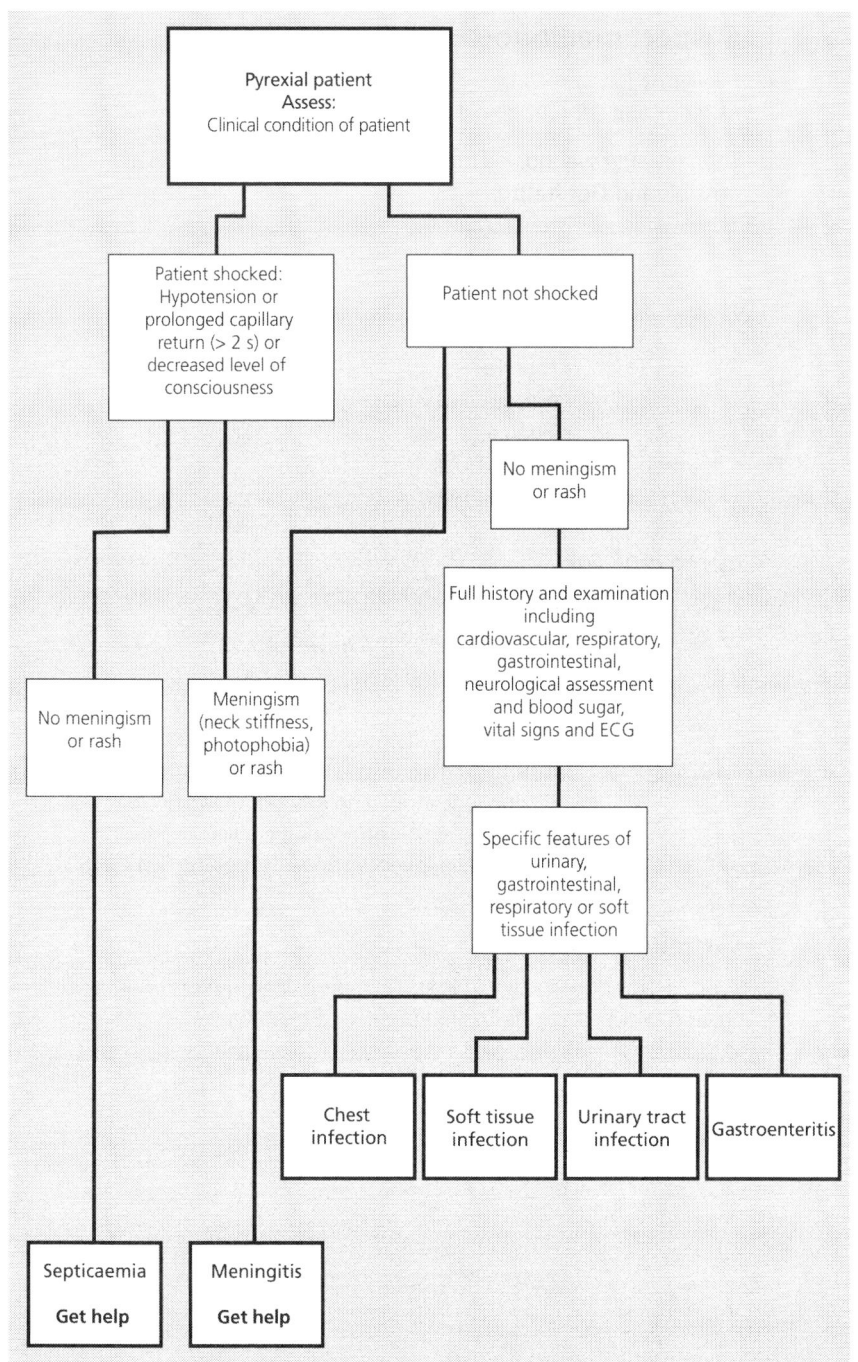

```
                    Pyrexial patient
                       Assess:
              Clinical condition of patient
                    /            \
   Patient shocked:              Patient not shocked
   Hypotension or                        |
   prolonged capillary            No meningism
   return (> 2 s) or                 or rash
   decreased level of                    |
   consciousness                 Full history and examination
     /        \                         including
                                 cardiovascular, respiratory,
  No meningism   Meningism           gastrointestinal,
    or rash    (neck stiffness,    neurological assessment
               photophobia)           and blood sugar,
                 or rash            vital signs and ECG
                                          |
                                  Specific features of
                                       urinary,
                                   gastrointestinal,
                                  respiratory or soft
                                   tissue infection
                                  /    |    |    \
                             Chest  Soft tissue  Urinary tract  Gastroenteritis
                           infection  infection    infection
     |            |
  Septicaemia   Meningitis
  Get help      Get help
```

Meningococcal disease

> **Suspect meningococcal disease if:**
> - Fever AND
> - Meningism OR non-blanching rash
>
> Then give intravenous ceftriaxone 2 g (adult dose) as soon as possible and **Get help**

What to ask

- Feverish
- Nausea and vomiting
- Headache
- Photophobia
- Neck stiffness

What to look for

- Pyrexia
- Neck stiffness – not always present
- Altered mental state
- Photophobia
- Rash – particularly if non-blanching
- Kernig's sign (positive if headache increases on flexing legs at hip and extending at knee)
- Signs of shock – prolonged capillary refill, tachycardia, hypotension – if present **Get help**

> **Capillary refill**
> A good sign of early shock. Press on a digit, sternum or forehead for 5 s and release – capillary refill should occur within 2 s

MEDICAL

Investigations

- FBC, U&E's, glucose, coagulation screen, blood cultures (don't delay antibiotic until after cultures taken)
- Swabs (nasopharyngeal/skin rash) can be taken once initial management completed

Management

- Give high-flow oxygen
- Antibiotics (see above)
- Insert two large-bore cannulae – give IV fluids rapidly and reassess frequently
- All patients should be referred to a physician

Septic shock

> Septic shock is the combination of infection with signs of shock – prolonged capillary return, tachycardia, hypotension, altered mental state – if present **Get help** early

What to ask

- Recent / current illness
  - diarrhoea +/- vomiting
  - cough
  - urinary symptoms/presence of catheter
  - pelvic pain/vaginal discharge
- Recent injuries or burns
- Joint pain or swelling
- If currently menstruating whether using tampons
- Immunocompromised, eg steroid use, IV drug abuser, diabetes

What to look for

- Signs of shock – prolonged capillary return, tachycardia, hypotension, altered mental state
- Pyrexia
- Skin for
  - rash – if non-blanching see meningococcal disease (page 44-45)
  - erythema/abscess
  - recent burns or injuries

Investigations

- Capillary blood glucose – if low **treat immediately**
- FBC, U&E's, glucose, coagulation screen, blood cultures and other tests dependent on possible cause
- ECG
- Chest X-ray

MEDICAL

Management

- Get help immediately
- Give high-flow oxygen
- Hypoglycaemia – 50–150 ml of 20% dextrose IV or 1 mg of glucagon IM (may not work in alcoholics)
- Insert two large-bore cannulae – give IV fluids rapidly and reassess frequently
- Broad spectrum IV antibiotics
- All patients should be referred to a physician

My department's policy for antibiotics in septic shock:

Urinary tract infection (UTI)

What to ask

- Dysuria
- Frequency
- Haematuria
- Abdominal/back pain
- Systemic upset (nausea and vomiting, malaise, rigors)

What to look for

- Pyrexia
- Suprapubic tenderness
- Loin tenderness
- Signs of shock – prolonged capillary return, tachycardia, hypotension, altered mental state – if present **Get help**

Investigations

If patient is systemically well and there are no signs of shock:
- Urinalysis
- Urine microscopy – if equivocal findings on urinalysis but history very suggestive of infection
- Capillary blood glucose

If patient is systemically unwell or signs of shock:
- FBC, U&E's, glucose
- Blood cultures

Differential diagnoses

- Sexually transmitted infections – may cause urinary symptoms. Ask about urethral/vaginal discharge and any symptoms in partner. Refer to Genitourinary Medicine clinic if suspected

Management

- Encourage fluids
- Analgesia and antibiotics

MEDICAL

Who to admit

- Patients who are systemically unwell particularly if vomiting
- Patients with signs of shock
- Patients who are elderly and 'off feet' **or** disorientated **or** there is poor home support

My department's UTI antibiotic policy:

ILLNESS

Gastroenteritis

> Don't forget infection control – wash your hands after dealing with the patient. Gastroenteritis is very contagious – you don't want it and neither do all your other patients

What to ask

- Vomiting and/or diarrhoea
- Blood in vomit/stool
- Foreign travel
- Any suspicion of food poisoning

What to look for

- Pyrexia
- Signs of dehydration – dry mucous membranes, reduced urine output, lethargy
- Signs of shock – prolonged capillary return, tachycardia, hypotension, altered mental state – if present **Get help**
- Urine output
- Signs of peritonism – involuntary guarding, rebound tenderness

Investigations

- In severe illness or shock – FBC, U&E's, glucose
- Stool sample for culture and sensitivity

Management

- IV fluids – 1 l of saline over 1 h can make a weary patient feel much better and able to be sent home
- Antibiotics should only be given if the organism is known and treatment is recommended
- Avoid anti-diarrhoeals and antiemetics
- Food poisoning is a notifiable disease (find out your department's policy on notifying)

MEDICAL

Who to admit

- Any patient with bloody diarrhoea/haematemesis
- Any patient with signs of shock/severe dehydration
- Elderly patients with anything more than mild symptoms
- Any patient with anything more than mild symptoms and no home support

---

Other causes of diarrhoea and/or vomiting
- Constipation
- Bowel obstruction
- Inflammatory bowel disease
- Appendicitis
- Many infectious diseases

The patient with infection – diagnosis uncertain

If no cause can be found for a pyrexia check

- Signs of shock – prolonged capillary return, tachycardia, hypotension, altered mental state – if present **Get help**
- Look at whole of body for evidence of skin infection
- If recent travel abroad
  - in malaria endemic area – send blood for thick and thin film
  - if malaria not possible – consider simple illnesses (eg flu) as well as tropical illness
- If patient is known to be immunocompromised, eg malignancy, IV drug abuse, look for atypical and occult infections such as tuberculosis
- If possibility that ecstasy has been taken – **Get help**

Refer to a physician, all pyrexial patients:

- Known to be neutropoenic
- Post-splenectomy
- With sickle cell disease

Refer to a physician, patients with a fever and no obvious source if:

- Elderly and are disorientated or have poor home support
- Fever has been prolonged (ie > 48h)
- Diabetic and poor glycaemic control

Rarer causes for fever
- Malignancy – eg leukaemia/lymphoma
- Metabolic – thyrotoxicosis/Addison's disease
- Environmental – heat stroke/heat exhaustion

MEDICAL

Diabetes mellitus
Hypoglycaemia

Blood sugar below 3 mmol/l, usually occurs in diabetics

What to ask

- History of diabetes mellitus
- Recent change in diabetic medication regime
- Missed meals, vomiting or excessive exercise
- Excess alcohol or known liver disease

What to look for

- Sweating, tachycardia or blurred vision
- Decreased conscious level, drowsiness, fitting or violent behaviour – **Get help**

Investigations

- Capillary blood glucose
- FBC, U&E's, glucose. Take these once initial treatment has been given

Management

- If patient able, give oral glucose drink
- Dextrose IV – 50–100 ml of 20% dextrose
- Glucagon – 1 mg IV or IM
- Repeat capillary blood glucose

Who needs referral

- If no cause found or due to intercurrent illness, eg gastroenteritis, refer to on-call physicians
- If recovered and cause found, eg missed meal, then discharge with GP/diabetic team follow-up
- If remains drowsy with normal capillary blood sugar then look for another cause of decreased level of consciousness

ILLNESS

Hyperglycaemia

Diabetic ketoacidosis is a much more common cause than hyperosmolar non-ketotic hyperglycaemia (HONK). In older people with high capillary blood sugar but no ketones suspect HONK and **Get help**

What to ask

- Previous history of diabetes mellitus or symptoms of diabetes, eg polyuria, polydypsia and weight loss
- Missed insulin medications
- Recent illness, eg infections

What to look for

- Decreased conscious level, drowsiness, fitting or violent behaviour – **Get help**
- Shock, tachycardia, prolonged capillary refill or hypotensive – **Get help**

Investigations

- Capillary blood glucose
- FBC, U&E's, glucose, arterial blood gases and blood cultures; take these once initial treatment has been commenced
- Urinalysis
- Chest X-ray looking for focus of infection
- ECG

Management

- IV Normal saline (0.9%), at least 20 ml/kg in the first hour, these patients need fluid first of all (if suspect HONK use 0.45% saline)
- Insulin – 10 units (eg Actrapid or Humulin S) IV followed by sliding scale
- Monitor capillary blood glucose closely
- Strict fluid balance charting

MEDICAL 55

Who needs referral

- Refer all to on-call physicians

My department's protocol for sliding scale is:

ILLNESS

56 ILLNESS

Headache
Headache flowchart

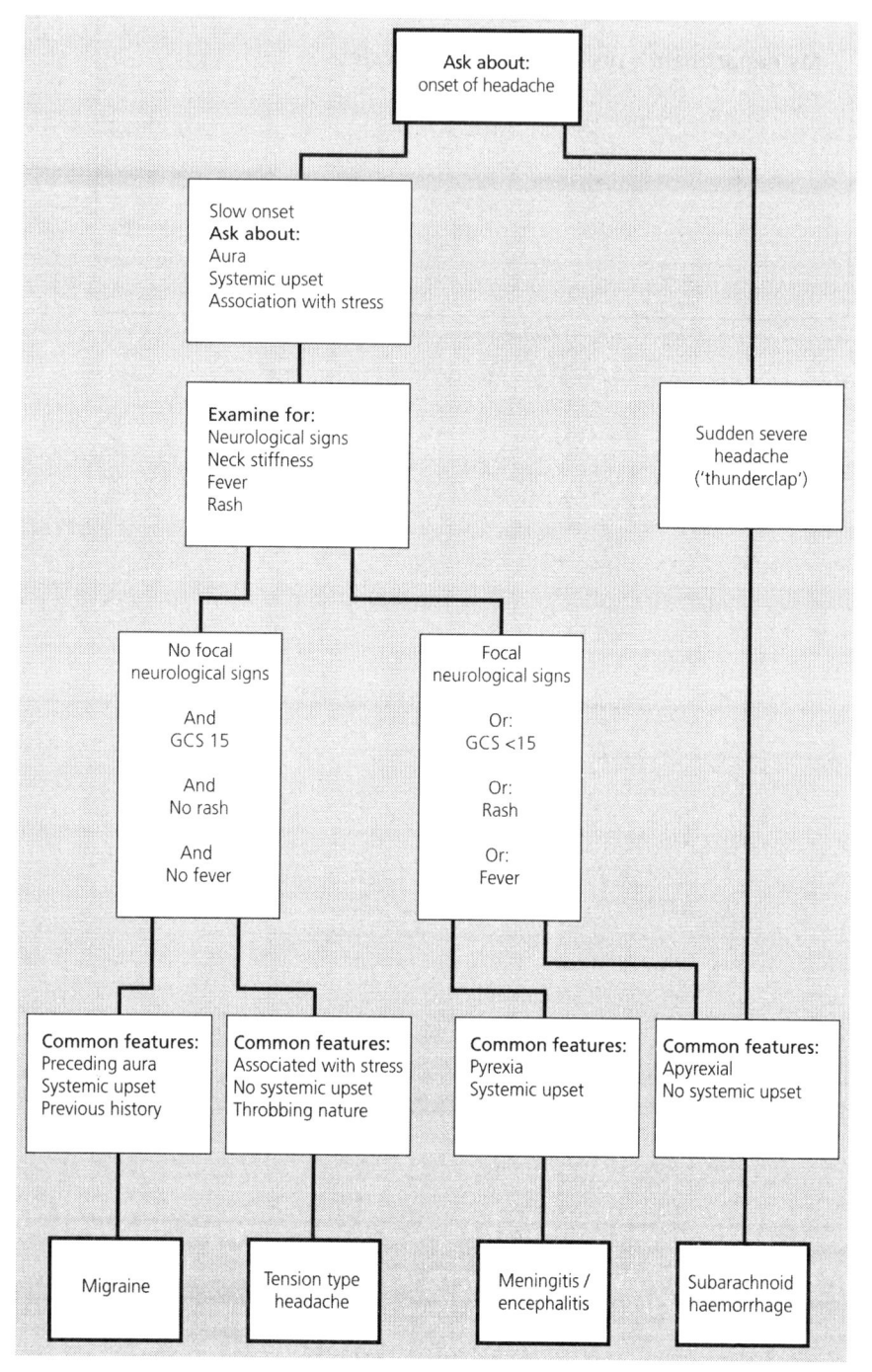

```
                        Ask about:
                     onset of headache
                    /                  \
        Slow onset                      Sudden severe
        Ask about:                      headache
        Aura                            ('thunderclap')
        Systemic upset
        Association with stress
                |
        Examine for:
        Neurological signs
        Neck stiffness
        Fever
        Rash
            /        \
    No focal          Focal
    neurological      neurological
    signs             signs
    And               Or:
    GCS 15            GCS <15
    And               Or:
    No rash           Rash
    And               Or:
    No fever          Fever
```

Common features:	Common features:	Common features:	Common features:
Preceding aura	Associated with stress	Pyrexia	Apyrexial
Systemic upset	No systemic upset	Systemic upset	No systemic upset
Previous history	Throbbing nature		

| Migraine | Tension type headache | Meningitis / encephalitis | Subarachnoid haemorrhage |

MEDICAL

Subarachnoid haemorrhage

What to ask

- Sudden severe onset of headache ('like being hit on back of head')
- Association with exercise/sexual activity/stimulant drugs
- Past history of hypertension
- Drug history – anticoagulants
- Family history of subarachnoid haemorrhage

What to look for

- Reduced level of consciousness/fitting – **Get help**
- Focal neurological signs
- Hypertension
- Neck stiffness
- Rarely retinal haemorrhages subhyaloid (blood between retina and vitreous)

Investigations

- FBC, U&E's, coagulation screen, glucose, group and save
- ECG – may show variety of abnormalities
- Get advice regarding your department's policy on further investigation
- Give adequate analgesia
- Refer all patients to a physician or neurosurgeon dependent on local policy

---

Headache associated with sexual activity
(after or during, not before)

Often patients too embarrassed to reveal. May be a variant of a migraine headache but also may be subarachnoid bleed. Differentiation is usually impossible and patient should be referred for further investigation.

ILLNESS

Migraine

What to ask

- Is this an exacerbation of a pre-existing problem or a possible new diagnosis
  - If known migraine sufferer:
    Usual migraine symptoms/frequency
    Normal medication
    What is different about this episode
  - If not known migraine sufferer:
    Presence of aura/systemic symptoms, eg nausea, visual disturbance
- Onset – if sudden and severe *see* subarachnoid haemorrhage (page 57)
- It is rare for migraine to first present above the age of 25

What to look for

- There should be no neurological abnormality, temperature or rash
- Check blood pressure

Management

- Start with simple analgesics and antiemetic, eg paracetamol 1 g, ibuprofen 400 mg and metoclopramide 10 mg
- Keep in quiet, dark room and review within an hour
- If not settling or already tried simple analgesia consider a triptan, eg sumatriptan orally/subcutaneous/nasal spray – check contraindication to use
- Avoid a triptan if already taking ergotamine prophylaxis

Who needs referral

- If intractable or severe despite treatment

MEDICAL

If you are discharging the patient, advise:

- A quiet restful environment
- Drink plenty of fluids
- Return if not settling or worsens
- Make an appointment to see the GP for further management

ILLNESS

Headache – diagnosis uncertain

Always check

- Presence of neurological signs – particularly papilloedema – although very rare
- Blood pressure – malignant hypertension may cause headache
- If there is temporal/occipital tenderness in any patient over 50, which may signify giant cell arteritis
- Presence of rash, meningism or pyrexia – *see* Meningococcal disease page 44-45

Giant cell arteritis

- May cause visual disturbance
- Is often associated with joint aching and myalgia
- The ESR is usually raised > 50

If giant cell arteritis is possible, discuss with senior or a physician

---

Always refer headache patients with

- Severe headache – 'the worst headache ever'
- Any neurological signs, confusion or disorientation
- Early morning headaches
- Meningism

Headaches are rarely caused by

- Eye refractive errors – advising patients to get their eyes checked is rarely appropriate and can delay definitive diagnosis
- Sinus disease – usually other signs are present, eg localised tenderness/fever

Other causes of headache

- **Neck spondylitis** – check if movement of neck exacerbates headache but beware neck stiffness is associated with subarachnoid haemorrhage and meningitis
- **Raised intracranial pressure** – typically early morning headache worse on coughing/straining
- **Cluster headache** – unilateral severe pain concentrated around the eye. Associated with watering of eye/running of nose. Usually occurs at same time of day – often at night
- **Carbon monoxide** – consider if several members of family unwell or if headache is associated with use of heating particularly old or unserviced boilers
- **Nitrate-induced** – headache occurs after using spray or taking medication

Poisoning

Overdose

This is a basic overview of managing a patient who has taken an overdose. The patient could have taken a number of medications and/or street drugs. Often the history will be unreliable or the patient may be too unwell to give a history.

What to ask

- What substance and quantity was taken
- Time of ingestion
- Was alcohol taken with the substance
- Accidental or suicidal intent
- Past history of self-harm or overdose
- Have they vomited since

What to look for

- Is the patient able to maintain their airway, if compromised **Get help**
- GCS and pupil size and reaction
- Agitation and restlessness
- Blood capillary glucose and temperature
- Injection sites

Investigations

- FBC, U&E's, coagulation screen, LFT, paracetamol and salicylate levels
- ABG if suggested by TOXBASE
- Chest X-ray if vomited – aspiration?
- ECG if suggested by TOXBASE

Management

- Mostly depends on the substance taken. Always consult TOXBASE or contact the poisons information centre for appropriate treatment
- If hypoglycaemic give 50–100 ml of 20% dextrose

MEDICAL

- Remember that these patients may deteriorate very quickly

Who to admit

- As advised by TOXBASE
- Patients will need a psychiatric assessment when medically fit

TOXBASE website: www.spib.axl.co.uk

My department's number for Poisons information:

ILLNESS

ILLNESS

Paracetamol overdose

What to ask

- Time of overdose and quantity taken
- Any symptoms: nausea and vomiting, abdominal pain

Identify the patient at high risk of severe liver damage:
- Excess alcohol intake
- Liver disease
- Malnutrition
- HIV positive
- Enzyme inducing drugs

What to look for

- There are usually no physical signs
- If late presentation (more than 48 h), may be signs of hepatic failure

Investigations

- Paracetamol and salicylate (P/S) levels at 4 h post-ingestion or immediately if patient presents more than 4 h after ingestion
- FBC, U&E's, LFT, coagulation screen, glucose if more than 8 h since ingestion

Management

- Give 50 g charcoal if the patient presents within 1 h of ingestion
- Aim to treat with *N*-acetylcysteine (NAC) within 8 h of ingestion, this may mean starting it before the levels have come back
- Treat according to the paracetamol treatment normogram available in the BNF – check you are using the correct treatment line

MEDICAL

• Some patients develop an allergic reaction to NAC; STOP infusion and seek advice

NAC treatment schedule
- 150 mg/kg in 200 ml of 5% dextrose over 15 min
- 50 mg/kg in 500 ml of 5% dextrose over 4 h
- 100 mg/kg in 1000 ml of 5% dextrose over 16 h

Management dilemmas

- The P/S level is not back within 8 h: start treatment and stop if necessary when the results come back
- The patent presents later than 8 h after ingestion: start treatment immediately if significant overdose, eg > 12 g or 150 mg/kg
- The patient presents > 24 h post-ingestion – **Get help**
- The patient has taken a staggered overdose – P/S levels are unhelpful, it is usually better to treat with NAC
- If ever in doubt – treat!

Who to admit

- Any patient requiring treatment, refer to physician or manage on the observation ward
- Any patient not requiring admission needs a psychiatric assessment. Find out your department's policy for this

If patient was treated with NAC, the INR, creatinine and LFTs must be checked before discharge

ILLNESS

ILLNESS

Opiate overdose

Beware of co-proxamol, which contains dextropropoxyphene – this can cause life-threatening complications.

What to look for

- Respiratory depression
- Reduced level of conciousness
- Pinpoint pupils
- Venepuncture marks – has the patient injected? (arms, groin and neck are the most commonly used sites intravenous drug abusers (IVDAs))

Complications
- Hypothermia
- Hypotension
- Arrhythmias
- Pulmonary oedema
- Convulsions
- Renal failure

Investigations

- If complications or GCS<9 – **Get help**
- FBC, U&E's, P/S, coagulation screen, blood glucose

Management

- High-flow oxygen
- Naloxone 0.8 mg IV, repeat if necessary to a maximum of 10 mg
- Beware that naloxone has a short duration of action and coma or respiratory depression can recur – don't walk away!
- If you need to consider an infusion of naloxone – **Get help**
- Monitor, give naloxone little and often; cardiac arrest is possible with reversal

MEDICAL

Who to admit

- All for observation
- Many IVDAs will attempt to leave; if this is a possibility give 0.8 mg naloxone IM and try to persuade them to stay

Tricyclic antidepressant overdose

Patients who have taken a significant overdose may be unable to give you a history. Symptoms occur within 4 h of ingestion. **Get help early**

What to look for

- Anticholinergic effects: dry mouth, blurred vision, tachycardia, dilated pupils
- In severe overdose signs include: coma, convulsions, hypotension and arrhythmias –
Get help

Investigations

- Consult TOXBASE
- Capillary blood glucose
- FBC, U&E's, glucose, paracetamol and salicylate levels
- ABG
- ECG: sinus tachycardia, widening of QRS complex, variety of arrhythmias including broad complex tachycardia

Management

- Mainly supportive
- High-flow oxygen
- Maintain airway; intubation may be required.
Get help
- Give sodium bicarbonate 1 mmol/kg of 8.4% if ECG abnormalities or acidosis on ABG
- Treat convulsions with IV lorazepam 2–4 mg

Who to admit

- ALL!

MEDICAL

Severe allergic reaction

This is an emergency. Treatment may need to be commenced while taking a history. **Get help** if signs of an airway problem.

What to ask

- Onset of allergic reaction
- Known allergens
- Any new medications, food, recent vaccination
- Bee/wasp sting
- Any difficulty breathing

What to look for

- Signs of shock – prolonged capillary refill, tachycardia, hypotension – **Get help**
- Bronchospasm
- Angioedema
- Cough, erythema, pruritus, urticaria, nausea, vomiting

Management

- STOP any current infusions
- High-flow oxygen
- If unconscious, place in recovery position
- If signs of shock, **Get help** and give 0.5 ml of 1:1000 IM adrenaline immediately (can be repeated every 5–10 min)
- Insert two large-bore cannulae and give IV fluids rapidly and reassess
- Give 10 mg IV chlorpheniramine and 200 mg IV hydrocortisone

---

- Patients on beta-blockers may be resistant to adrenaline and require a glucagon infusion
- 20% of patients will have a repeat reaction 4–8 h after the initial event

---

Who to admit

- All patients should be referred to the physician on call

ILLNESS

Thromboembolic problems
Deep vein thrombosis (DVT)

Always enquire about symptoms of pulmonary embolus (PE, see page 26–27) and beware, a missed DVT could result in a PE

What to ask

- Site of pain or tenderness
- Duration of tenderness
- Any chest pain, breathlessness or haemoptysis
- Risk factors: surgery, immobility, long flights, pregnancy, oral contraceptive pill, hormone replacement therapy, malignancy, previous thromboembolic problems
- Family history of thromboembolic problems

What to look for

- Swelling, erthyema, warmth and tenderness (these signs will be distal to the occlusion)
- Homan's sign: dorsiflexion of the foot may cause pain, however is not a reliable sign
- There may be no clinical signs in the presence of a DVT

Differential diagnosis

- Ruptured Baker's cyst
- Muscle tear
- Superficial thrombophlebitis

Investigations

- Measure the limb, significant swelling is defined as 2 cm difference between the two sides
- D-dimer
- Doppler ultrasound or venogram (gold standard)
- If necessary investigate on clinical suspicion alone

MEDICAL

Management

> My department's policy for LMWH (low molecular weight heparin):

Who to admit

- All patients should be discussed with a senior or the physician on-call

Environmental problems
Hypothermia
What to ask

- Has the patient been exposed to cold temperature or cold water
- Ingestion of drugs or alcohol
- Recent illness, particularly the old/young
- Trauma
- Known endocrine problems

Investigations

- Be careful when moving your patient as it may precipitate ventricular fibrillation
- Rectal temperature
- Blood capillary glucose
- FBC, U&E's, glucose, amylase, thyroid function tests
- ABG: respiratory or metabolic acidosis
- Chest X-ray

MEDICAL

	Mild 32–35°C	Moderate/severe <32°C
Look for	• Shivering (absent below 32°C) • Tachypnoea	• Confusion/reduced GCS • Bradycardia • Hypotension • ↓Respiratory rate • Arrhythmias
Management	• Remove wet clothes • Cover with warming blankets • Warm room • Humidified oxygen • Warm fluids IV	• As for mild, however **Get help** Further treatment may be required • Beware not to overload the elderly with fluid! • If VF arrest, may not respond to defibrillation below 30°C, continue CPR until at least 35°C
Referral	Discharge if no underlying medical problem, complications and social circumstances adequate	Refer to physicians

ILLNESS

Haematological problems
Sickle cell anaemia (SCA)

What to ask
- Known to have SCA or family history
- Site of pain (typically severe pain – can be anywhere)
- Recent infection, exposure to cold, dehydration
- Possible pregnancy

What to look for
- Chest syndrome: pleuritic chest pain, dyspnoea, tachypnoea
- Abdominal syndrome: abdominal pain but no peritonism, vomiting, jaundice
- Neurological deficit – CVA, convulsions
- Pyrexia
- Priapism
- Bone pain and/or swelling if hands/feet
- If signs of shock: prolonged capillary refill, tachycardia, hypotension – **Get help**

Investigations
- FBC, U&E's, reticulocyte count, amylase, glucose, group and save, blood cultures
- ABG: if $PO_2 < 9$ **Get help**
- Chest X-ray
- ECG

Management
- High-flow oxygen
- Warm blankets
- Titrate IV morphine or diamorphine for analgesia and give antiemetic
- Insert two large-bore cannulae and give 1 l IV fluid over 3 h (reduces viscosity)
- Antibiotics according to your hospital's policy

MEDICAL

> **The patient will often know the best management for themselves. Treat early to avoid complications**

> **My department's policy on antibiotics for SCA:**

Who to admit

- Discuss all patients with a senior physician on-call or haematologist

Psychiatry

Mental state health examination

You cannot expect to take a detailed history that normally takes a psychiatrist an hour. However, on referral you must have assessed the patient adequately and this includes a mental state examination.

Appearance

- How are they dressed: dirty clothes, drunk, tremor

Behaviour

- Aggressive, hostile, quiet, nervous, tense
- Eye contact

Speech

- Quantity, rate, rhythm, articulate, muddled
- Jumping from one subject to another (flight of ideas)

Mood

- Subjective and objective; angry, irritable, happy; ask about eating, sleeping habits, concentration, memory; self opinion

Thoughts

- Suicidal or depressive thoughts; preoccupations; abnormal beliefs or experiences; auditory or visual hallucinations; obsessions; feelings of guilt

Interaction with yourself

- Eye contact; co-operative; humorous; confident or shy

MEDICAL

Cognition

- Estimate the patient's cognitive function; mini mental state examination

Insight

- Is the patient aware of his/her problems and do they understand the need to accept them?

ILLNESS

ILLNESS

The suicidal/self-harm patient

Your patient may present with the same story every week or may be attending for the first time. Treat them the same and never be dismissive – you are bound to be caught out!

The crucial part of treating this patient is the assessment:
- Find a suitable room; take someone with you or ensure that there are appropriate facilities, eg panic button, two exits
- Gain the patient's trust
- Keep them calm
- Listen as much as possible

The assessment

- Suicidal ideas
- Known psychiatric disorder
- Factors associated with increased risk
- Social support
- Previous suicide attempts
- Mental state examination

Factors of increased suicide risk
- Male
- Divorced/single
- Unemployed
- Lack of support
- Chronic medical illness
- Psychiatric illness

Suicidal ideation

You need to establish the following:
- Do they still want to die / self harm?
- Why did they attempt suicide / self-harm?
- Was it a spontaneous action or carefully planned?

Who to admit

- Discuss all patients with a member of the on-call psychiatric team

MEDICAL

The agitated patient

The agitated person may be difficult to get a history from and may be violent. If you suspect that they may be violent always take a chaperone with you and make a senior member of staff in the department aware.

You cannot assume agitation has a psychiatric cause. Look for medical problems!

Possible medical causes of agitation

- Drug intoxication
- Infection
- Hypo-/hyperglycaemia
- Hypoxia
- Post-ictal
- Metabolic disorder
- Cerebral problem/head injury
- Distended bladder (common in the elderly)

Features helpful in differentiating organic from psychiatric problems

	Organic	Psychiatric
Course	Fluctuating	Stable
Previous psychiatric history	Uncommon	Common
Vital signs	Abnormal	Normal
Orientation	Impaired	Occasionally impaired
Speech	Pressured / incoherent	Usually coherent
Hallucinations	Visual	Auditory

What to do

- Full examination and history, where possible, to rule out organic problem
- Investigations as appropriate to clinical findings
- For all patients, capillary blood glucose and oxygen saturation

continues overleaf

ILLNESS

ILLNESS

Your patient may have a psychiatric problem; however, the psychiatrist is often reluctant to see the patient unless an organic cause has been excluded

What if my patient is medically fit yet remains agitated and difficult to control?

- Drug treatment is an option but should only be used as a last resort as it may mask an underlying problem. **Get help**

My department's policy for sedation of the agitated patient:

MEDICAL

Alcohol problems

Your aim is to rule out any serious medical or psychiatric problems that may need treating. Some patients will just be looking for a bed for the night!

What to ask

- Amount and type of alcohol drunk
- Pattern of drinking (binge or regular intake)
- Time of day that the first drink is needed
- Withdrawal symptoms (shakes, nausea, agitation, irritability, sweating)

CAGE

Do you:
- Feel you should **cut** down on your drinking
- Get **annoyed** if other people mention your drinking
- Feel **guilty** about drinking
- Need an **eye-opener**

What to look for

Examine the patient. As a result of their alcohol intake they may have a serious medical problem that needs treating:

- Head injury (see page 146–147)
- Epileptic fit (see page 40–41)
- Pancreatitis (see page 92–93)
- Hypoglycaemia (see page 53)
- Intercurrent infection (see page 52)
- Acute withdrawal
- Delirium tremens (tremors, hallucinations, sweating, fits, tachycardia). **This is a medical emergency. Get help**

continues overleaf

ILLNESS

ILLNESS

Investigations

- FBC, blood capillary glucose, FBC, mean cell volume, gamma-GT, LFT, amylase

Management

- Rehydrate with iv fluids if unwell
- Pabrinex® 2 pairs, tds if being admitted

Who to admit

The patient may be sent home if they have no medical or psychiatric problem, are conscious, able to walk and are preferably with an able adult
- If medically unwell
- If medically fit; however, if you are concerned they may be a danger to themselves or others discuss with the psychiatrist
- Inform GP in all cases

Local alcohol support number:

MEDICAL

Refusal of treatment

Dealing with a patient who refuses treatment is always difficult. This is a basic guideline. Always:
- Seek advice from your senior or a psychiatrist
- Document everything
- Obtain a witness to events if possible

What to do

- Assess the capacity of the patient
  - The patient must be able to **understand** and **retain** information regarding the treatment, its benefits, risks and the consequences of not having the treatment
  - The patient must **believe** that information
  - The patient must be capable of weighing up the information in order to arrive at a conclusion, ie **evaluate**

What if the patient is not deemed to be competent?

- Ask for a psychiatric opinion. If thought to have an underlying psychiatric problem, the patient can be detained under the Mental Health Act. The patient can then be treated for a medical problem BUT only under the direction of the psychiatrist

What if the patient leaves the Emergency Department in the meantime?

- You may ask the Police to return them if they are likely to come to significant harm

What if the patient proves to be competent, yet still refuses treatment?

- Discuss with a senior, even if this is the Consultant at home.

ILLNESS

Ophthalmology
Visual problems/painful eye

What to ask

- If eye has been injured see Eye injury (see page 152–153)
- If no injury ask about:
  - Pain in the eye
  - Discharge from the eye
  - Alteration in vision
  - Previous eye problems

What to look for

- All patients must have their visual acuity checked – see Eye injury (see page 152–153) for further details
- If the patient is unable to keep their eye open for examination use local anaesthetic drops
- Use fluorescein drops and look for uptake (shows green with a blue light to indicate damage to the epithelium)
- Check for:
  - Conjunctival redness – localised or generalised
  - Corneal ulceration – uptake of fluorescein
  - Retinal changes if any visual loss or disturbance

Management

- Visual loss – any patient with total or partial visual loss (including 'curtain coming down' or 'flashes of light') should be referred to an ophthalmologist
- Acute glaucoma – associated with severe eye pain, visual disturbance and a fixed mid-sized pupil. If suspected discuss with a senior or an ophthalmologist

MEDICAL

Common eye problems

- **Conjunctivitis** – itchiness, watering and discharge from the eye. The conjunctiva is generally red. Take a swab in neonates for chlamydia and gonococcus. Treat with antibiotic eye ointment
- **Arc eye** – exposure to welding/sun lamp. General conjunctival redness and photophobia. Treat with antibiotic ointment and analgesia
- **Corneal ulcer** – localised or generalised conjunctival injection and fluorescein uptake on cornea. Refer all to ophthalmologist
- **Contact lens lost in eye** – fluorescein may help to localise. If unable to find – discuss with a senior or ophthalmologist

Chapter 2
SURGERY

ILLNESS

88 ILLNESS

Abdominal pain
Abdominal pain flowchart

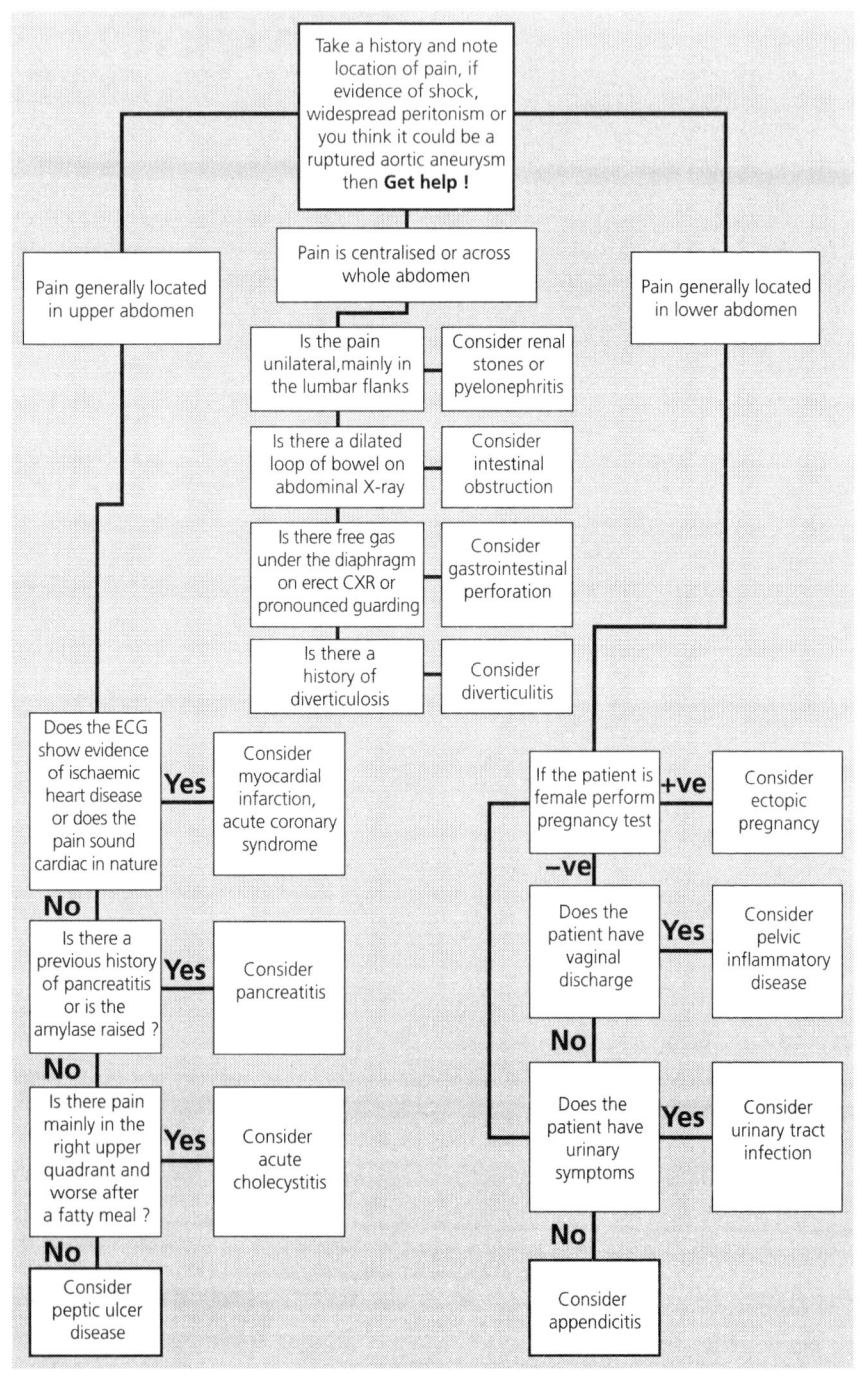

Take a history and note location of pain, if evidence of shock, widespread peritonism or you think it could be a ruptured aortic aneurysm then **Get help !**

Pain is centralised or across whole abdomen

- Is the pain unilateral, mainly in the lumbar flanks → Consider renal stones or pyelonephritis
- Is there a dilated loop of bowel on abdominal X-ray → Consider intestinal obstruction
- Is there free gas under the diaphragm on erect CXR or pronounced guarding → Consider gastrointestinal perforation
- Is there a history of diverticulosis → Consider diverticulitis

Pain generally located in upper abdomen

- Does the ECG show evidence of ischaemic heart disease or does the pain sound cardiac in nature **Yes** → Consider myocardial infarction, acute coronary syndrome
- **No** ↓ Is there a previous history of pancreatitis or is the amylase raised ? **Yes** → Consider pancreatitis
- **No** ↓ Is there pain mainly in the right upper quadrant and worse after a fatty meal ? **Yes** → Consider acute cholecystitis
- **No** ↓ Consider peptic ulcer disease

Pain generally located in lower abdomen

- If the patient is female perform pregnancy test **+ve** → Consider ectopic pregnancy
- **–ve** ↓ Does the patient have vaginal discharge **Yes** → Consider pelvic inflammatory disease
- **No** ↓ Does the patient have urinary symptoms **Yes** → Consider urinary tract infection
- **No** ↓ Consider appendicitis

SURGERY

Ruptured abdominal aortic aneurysm

Commonly occurs in over 55 year olds but can present with varied symptoms so always consider this in anyone with abdominal **or** back pain. Often mistaken for Renal colic (see page 101).
If you suspect this then **Get help**

What to ask

- Location of pain specifically back pain
- Previous history of any vascular or cardiac disease
- Previous scans, often the patient is known to have an aneurysm and may even know the size of it

What to look for

- Pulsatile expansile mass is not always present, there may just be generalised tenderness
- Shock, tachycardia, prolonged capillary refill or hypotensive **Get help**
- Radio femoral delay
- Absent or very weak femoral pulses

Investigations

- Don't delay surgical referral for investigations, do them while you are waiting for help
- FBC, U&E's, blood glucose, coagulation screen, cross match 10 units of blood

Management

- **Get help**
- Refer to senior surgical/vascular on-call
- Give oxygen
- Two large-bore IV cannulae with fluids aiming for a systolic BP of around 90 mmHg (higher may cause faster leaking from the aneurysm)
- Small titrations of IV morphine/diamorphine for analgesia and give antiemetic
- Insert a urinary catheter

ILLNESS

ILLNESS

Intestinal obstruction

Usually this will be due to a physical blockage in the lumen, eg tumour, or something pressing on the lumen wall, eg adhesions or obstructed hernia.

What to ask

- Previous occurrences or any abdominal surgery (causing adhesions)
- Vomiting – early problem in upper GI obstruction
- Constipation (absolute if no flatus) – early problem in lower GI obstruction
- Known hernias
- About the pain – may be colicky in nature
- If they have noticed any increasing abdominal distension

> Always look for hernias including femoral hernias, as you can easily miss these whilst trying to 'protect the patient's modesty'

What to look for

- Signs of dehydration – dry mucous membranes, reduced urine output or lethargy
- Signs of shock: tachycardia, prolonged capillary refill or hypotensive – **Get help**
- Generalised abdominal tenderness
- Bowel sounds, high-pitched – early; absent – late

Investigations

- FBC, U&E's, amylase, glucose, group and save
- Abdominal X-ray showing dilated bowel
- Erect chest X-ray if perforation (see page 102) a possibility

SURGERY

Management

- IV fluids
- Titrate IV morphine/diamorphine for analgesia and give an antiemetic
- Keep nil by mouth and if vomiting arrange for a nasogastric tube to be passed
- Urinary catheter to measure fluid balance

Who needs referral

Refer all to surgical on-call team

ILLNESS

Pancreatitis

What to ask

- Location of the pain, specifically epigastric and if radiates into the upper back
- Previous occurrences
- Excess alcohol intake and gall stones (the most common risk factors)

What to look for

- Epigastric tenderness with localised or diffuse involuntary guarding and rebound tenderness
- Evidence of chronic alcohol use such as spider naevi and jaundice
- Signs of shock, tachycardia, prolonged capillary refill or hypotensive – **Get help**

Investigations

- FBC, U&E's, LFTs, amylase, calcium, glucose, ABG
- Chest X-ray
- ECG

> **In my hospital the upper limit for normal amylase is:**

Management

- Oxygen
- IV fluids
- Titrate IV morphine/diamorphine for analgesia and give an antiemetic
- Keep nil by mouth and if vomiting arrange for a nasogastric tube

Who needs referral?

- Refer all to surgical on-call team

Amylase can also be raised in:
- Perforated peptic ulcer
- Cholecystitis
- Intestinal obstruction
- Ruptured ectopic pregnancy

However remember amylase may not be raised in acute or chronic pancreatitis

Acute cholecystitis

Inflammation of the gall bladder or the biliary tree usually associated with gallstone.

What to ask

- Location of pain, occurs in the right upper quadrant and often radiates to the back
- If pain is associated with a large or fatty meal
- Nausea or vomiting

What to look for?

- Tenderness in the right upper quadrant, possibly with guarding, Murphy's sign positive
- Patients often are 'Fat, Forties, Fair, Fertile, Female'
- Pyrexia

How to perform Murphy's sign

Palpate the right upper quadrant under the costal margin. Ask the patient to breathe deeply and if they get sudden pain (as the gall bladder moves down) or guarding this is positive suggesting cholecystitis

Investigations

- FBC, blood glucose, U&E's, LFTs, amylase, blood cultures

Management

- Analgesia, usually titrate IV morphine/diamorphine for analgesia and give an antiemetic

Who needs referral?

- Refer all but those with mild fully resolved symptoms to on-call surgical doctor for assessment

SURGERY

If sending the patient home

- Fully resolved symptoms probably are due to biliary colic, not acute cholecystitis
- Ensure patient's understanding of their condition and their ability to return if pain recurs
- Ensure GP follow-up

Diverticulitis

Inflammation of a diverticulum. Diverticulosis (presence of diverticulae) is a common condition in the middle-aged and elderly usually only causing mild symptoms, rarely resulting in an acute presentation.

What to ask

- History of diverticulosis or alteration in bowel habit with passage of mucus and/or blood
- Dull lower abdominal or pelvic pain localised in the early stages
- Symptoms of intestinal obstruction or perforation

What to look for

- Signs of shock, tachycardia, prolonged capillary refill or hypotensive – **Get help**
- Localised or diffuse involuntary guarding and rebound tenderness
- Pyrexia

Investigations

- FBC, U&E's, glucose, blood cultures
- Erect chest X-ray looking for perforation and abdominal X-ray looking for obstruction

Management

- IV fluids
- Titrate IV morphine/diamorphine for analgesia and give an antiemetic

Who needs referral?

- Refer all to surgical on-call team

SURGERY

Pelvic inflammatory disease (PID)

Occurs in sexually active women, as it is a sexually transmitted infection that may affect any part of the reproductive system. If left untreated can result in infertility or ectopic pregnancies.

What to ask

- Lower abdominal pain
- Offensive vaginal discharge
- Altered menstrual cycle varying from intermenstrual bleeding to late menstruation

What to look for

- Localised or diffuse involuntary guarding and rebound tenderness
- Pyrexia
- Signs of shock, tachycardia, prolonged capillary refill or hypotensive – **Get help**

Investigations

- FBC, U&E's, glucose
- Urinalysis
- High vaginal swabs should be done if you know how or by on-call gynaecologist or senior

Management

- Analgesia dependent on severity of symptoms, NSAID eg ibuprofen 400 mg orally for mild discomfort or titrate IV morphine/diamorphine for analgesia and give an antiemetic

Who needs referral?

- Mild discomfort can be referred to GP or outpatient gynaecology clinic for results of investigations
- Any more than mild discomfort should be referred to gynaecology on call for further assessment

continues overleaf

ILLNESS

ILLNESS

My department's policy on antibiotics for PID:

SURGERY

Appendicitis

Most common cause of acute abdomen in the UK. Essentially a clinical diagnosis, usually under the age of 30 years

What to ask

- Central non-specific abdominal pain, may start in left iliac fossa and spread to the right
- Vomiting and anorexia
- Symptoms may be dependent on location of appendix

Varying location of appendix

- **Retrocaecal** – abdominal signs may be less obvious as behind the ascending colon
- **Pelvic** – may present with diarrhoea and have tenderness on PR examination or urinary symptoms

---

What to look for

- Initially there may be little to find and later there may be evidence of perforation
- Pyrexia, tachycardia, signs of dehydration – dry mucous membranes, reduced urine output or lethargy
- Tenderness in the right iliac fossa or on PR if pelvic appendix

Investigations

- Diagnosis is clinical!
- FBC to show raised white cell count but may still be normal in appendicitis

continues overleaf

ILLNESS

Management

- IV fluids
- Titrate IV morphine/diamorphine for analgesia and give an antiemetic
- Keep nil by mouth

Who needs referral?

- Refer all to surgical on-call team

SURGERY

Renal (ureteric) colic

This occurs because of clots or stones in the ureter. A ruptured aortic aneurysm (see page 89) can be mistaken for this common condition.

What to ask

- Usually there is a previous history of chronic renal disease or renal stones, but there's always a first time!
- Pain is severe but may be dull and consistent, it often comes in waves as the ureter tries to pass the stone down
- Pain often radiates to the external genitals (the same nerve supply as the trigone in the bladder)
- Frank (visible) haematuria
- Diuretic drugs

What to look for

- Loin and/or suprapubic tenderness usually only abdominal finding
- Pyrexia which may suggest associated urinary tract infection (see page 48–49)

Investigations

- Urinalysis shows haematuria in 90% of cases
- 'Kidney-ureter-bladder' (KUB) X-ray may show renal stones, look carefully down the tips of the lumbar spine processes where the ureters usually lie
- FBC, U&E's, glucose

Management

- Adequate analgesia, IV or IM NSAID according to local policy or titrate IV morphine/diamorphine and give an antiemetic (IM takes longer to act)

Who needs referral?

- Refer all first-time presentations to surgeons or urology on call
- If symptoms resolve in recurrent presentation ensure either GP or urologist follow-up

ILLNESS

Gastrointestinal perforation

What to ask

- May occur in patients with peptic ulcer disease, inflammatory bowel disease, gastrointestinal tumours
- Symptoms of obstruction, appendicitis, diverticulitis
- Severe abdominal pain which may have started very suddenly and might reduce initially in intensity with time

What to look for

- Tenderness initially localised in part of the abdomen and then becoming more generalised as it progresses
- Localised or diffuse involuntary guarding and rebound tenderness
- Absent bowel sounds
- Pyrexia:
- Signs of shock: tachycardia, prolonged capillary refill or hypotensive – **Get help**

Investigations

- FBC, U&E's, amylase, glucose, group and save
- Erect chest X-ray may show gas under the diaphragm (must sit up for around 10 min prior to X-ray)
- Abdominal X-ray may show free gas but can be difficult to interpret

Management

- **Get help**
- Give oxygen
- Titrate IV morphine/diamorphine for analgesia and give an antiemetic
- Keep nil by mouth

Who needs referral?

- Refer all to surgical on-call team

SURGERY

Abdominal pain – diagnosis uncertain

What must be done for all patients with abdominal pain

- Thorough history including previous surgery
- Examination including chest, abdomen, hernial orifices, rectal examination, genitalia
- Observations:
  - Pulse
  - Blood pressure
  - Oxygen saturation
  - Capillary blood glucose
- Urinalysis and pregnancy test

> Whilst 35% of cases of acute presentations are 'non-specific abdominal pain' this is a diagnosis of exclusion. Usually senior surgical doctors make it only after a period of observation on the ward with negative investigation results

Common mistakes in assessing abdominal pain

- Patient is now pain free but this may be due to analgesia and as this wears off the pain recurs
- Pregnancy not considered to prevent embarrassing questions, especially in adolescents with parents present
- Urinalysis not performed
- Not performing an ECG in epigastric pain and missing an inferior myocardial infarct

Other causes of abdominal pain to consider

- Peptic ulcer disease – very common condition with wide range of severity from mild heartburn to gastrointestinal perforation. Suggested by known peptic ulcer disease possibly with previous endoscopy. Recent NSAIDs, aspirin or steroids and excess alcohol consumption
- Abdominal malignancy – history of new dyspepsia in anyone over age 40 years should alert you to the

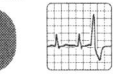

continues overleaf

ILLNESS

possibility of malignancy. Ask about weight loss, symptoms of metastases and family history.
- Gastroenteritis (see page 50–51)
- Diabetic ketoacidosis (see page 54–55)
- Irritable bowel syndrome
- Sickle cell disease (see page 74–75)
- Pneumonia (see page 22–23)

If you cannot find a cause for the patient's abdominal pain refer to on-call surgical doctor for observation and further investigation.

SURGERY

Acute arterial occlusion

What to ask

- Time since onset
- Past history of cardiovascular problems:
  - Atrial fibrillation
  - Heart valve disease
  - Intermittent claudication
  - TIA/CVA
  - Diabetes
- Drug history – warfarin / aspirin

What to look for

- The 6 'p's are a good guide:
  - **P**ulseless
  - **P**ainful
  - **P**allor
  - **P**araesthesia
  - **P**aralysis
  - **P**erishing cold
- Atrial fibrillation
- Heart murmurs
- Signs of shock – prolonged capillary refill, tachycardia, hypotension – if present **Get help**

Investigations

- FBC, U&E's, glucose, clotting screen, group and save serum
- ECG
- Chest X-ray

Management

- Give adequate analgesia – IV morphine and antiemetic are usually needed
- Refer **all** patients to a surgeon (preferably a vascular surgeon)

continues overleaf

Other conditions mimicking an acute arterial occlusion:

- **Shock / hypotension from another cause** – may produce pale, cold limbs if pre-existing vascular atherosclerotic disease
- **Massive iliofemoral DVT** – usually associated with a swollen cyanotic leg
- **Dissecting aortic aneurysm** – can cause acute arterial occlusion but normally associated with chest/back pain as well

SURGERY

Rectal bleeding
PR bleeding

What to ask

- Nature of bleeding – blood on wiping and sprayed around toilet bowl – suggests haemorrhoidal bleeding
- Pain – on defecation may indicate anal fissure
- Diarrhoea and vomiting – *see* gastroenteritis (page 50–51)
- Weight loss
- Past history of inflammatory bowel disease
- Drug history – NSAIDs/warfarin/steroids

What to look for

- Signs of shock – prolonged capillary refill, tachycardia, hypotension – if present **Get help**
- Abdominal signs – mass, tenderness, organomegaly
- Rectal examination – check for:
  - Blood
  - Anal fissure – tear in anal mucosa
  - Ulcer/mass

If bleeding from the upper GI tract is severe the patient may pass blood that is relatively unchanged.

Check for:
- Risk factors for peptic ulcer/oesophageal varices
- Upper abdominal tenderness

---

continues overleaf

ILLNESS

ILLNESS

Investigations

- FBC, U&E's, glucose, coagulation screen
- Group and save/cross match depending on clinical state – if shocked, cross match and order O-negative blood
- Abdominal X-ray if peritonism on examination

Management

- If significant bleeding, signs of shock or any abdominal findings, start IV fluids and refer to a surgeon

Patients can be discharged home if:

- Clear history of haemorrhoidal bleeding or anal fissure found on examination **and**
- No other cause for bleeding found on examination or investigation

SURGERY

Haematemesis and melaena

What to ask

- Estimated blood loss and over what period of time
- Any abdominal pain or previous occurrences
- Anticoagulants or NSAIDs
- Liver disease or alcohol abuse. If possible oesophageal varices then **Get help**
- Vomiting prior to haematemasis suggesting Mallory Weiss tear

What to look for

- Signs of shock: tachycardia, prolonged capillary refill or hypotensive – **Get help**
- Localised or diffuse involuntary guarding and rebound tenderness
- Altered blood in the rectum on PR examination
- Signs of chronic liver disease

Investigations

- FBC, U&E's, cross match 4 units if compromised (group and save if not)
- Chest X-ray for evidence of aspiration

Management

- IV fluids

Who needs referral?

- Refer all to on-call physician

Perianal abscess

What to ask

- Previous episodes
- Diabetes
- Inflammatory bowel disease
- Immunocompromised eg patient on steroids

What to look for

- Tenderness, swelling, erythema
- Discharge of pus
- Sinus in natal cleft – suggests pilonidal abscess
- Rectal examination is usually too painful to perform
- Signs of shock – prolonged capillary refill, tachycardia, hypotension – if present **Get help**

Investigations

- Capillary blood glucose
- FBC, U&E's, glucose, blood cultures if systemically unwell or known pre-existing problems, eg diabetes

Management

- Adequate analgesia – IV morphine and antiemetic may be needed
- Refer **all** patients to a surgeon

Don't be tempted to send someone home whose abscess appears to have already burst. A formal drainage procedure under general anaesthetic is usually needed to ensure that the abscess cavity is completely opened

SURGERY

Testicular pain
Testicular pain flowchart

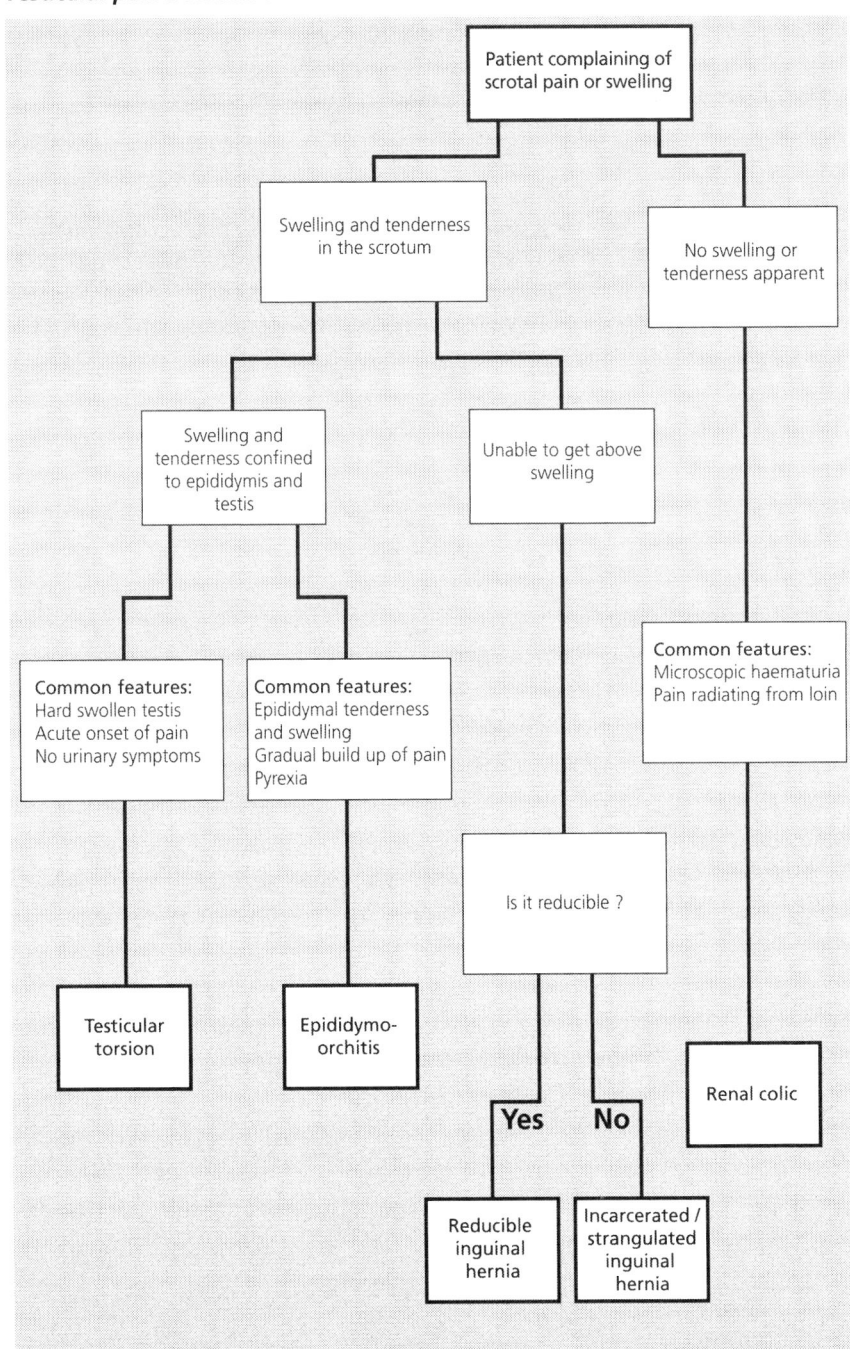

```
                    ┌─────────────────────┐
                    │ Patient complaining of │
                    │  scrotal pain or swelling │
                    └─────────────────────┘
                       │                │
          ┌────────────┘                └────────────┐
┌─────────────────────┐                   ┌─────────────────────┐
│ Swelling and tenderness │               │  No swelling or     │
│    in the scrotum       │               │  tenderness apparent │
└─────────────────────┘                   └─────────────────────┘
        │              │                            │
┌───────────────┐  ┌──────────────┐                 │
│ Swelling and  │  │ Unable to get │                │
│ tenderness    │  │ above swelling│                │
│ confined to   │  └──────────────┘                 │
│ epididymis and│                                   │
│ testis        │                        ┌─────────────────────┐
└───────────────┘                        │ Common features:    │
   │         │                           │ Microscopic haematuria│
                                         │ Pain radiating from loin│
                                         └─────────────────────┘
```

Common features:
Hard swollen testis
Acute onset of pain
No urinary symptoms

Common features:
Epididymal tenderness and swelling
Gradual build up of pain
Pyrexia

Is it reducible ?

Yes → Reducible inguinal hernia

No → Incarcerated / strangulated inguinal hernia

→ Testicular torsion

→ Epididymo-orchitis

→ Renal colic

Testicular torsion

> Testicular torsion is a surgical emergency –
> if suspected refer immediately to a surgeon

What to ask

- Time of onset
- Systemic upset – nausea and vomiting common
- Urinary symptoms – rare in torsion, think of alternate diagnosis
- Children may be shy and not disclose symptoms – be persistent

What to look for

- Swelling of hemiscrotum
- Exquisitely tender, hard testicle
- Sometimes reactive hydrocele may be found
- Some patients may have a mild pyrexia

Investigations

- Blood tests do not differentiate a torsion from another cause
- Don't delay referral for other tests, eg X-ray, ultrasound

Management

- Don't be tempted to try and manipulate the testis – this may make things a lot worse
- Refer **all** patients for a surgical/urology opinion

Epididymo-orchitis

What to ask

- Pain – usually gradual build up. May start in the flank or groin and spread to the scrotum
- Urinary symptoms are common
- Urethral discharge
- Sexual contacts
- Systemic upset

Causative organisms

- Coliforms – in prepubertal and >35 year olds
- Chlamydia and gonococcus – in young/middle aged

What to look for

- Epididymal swelling in early stages
- Testicular swelling later (epididymo-orchitis)
- Rectal examination for prostatitis – exquisite tenderness
- Pyrexia

Investigations

- FBC, U&E's, glucose – white cell count often high
- Urinalysis – only positive for infection in 25%

Management

- If testicular torsion cannot be excluded refer to a surgeon
- Antibiotics and follow-up according to your department's policy
- Adequate analgesia and scrotal support
- If possibility of sexually transmission advise follow-up in Genitourinary Medicine clinic for patient and partner, if known

continues overleaf

ILLNESS

> **My department's antibiotic regime for epididymo-orchitis:**

Who to admit

- Those who don't have satisfactory analgesia
- Those with significant systemic upset
- Those with evidence of an abscess – fluctuant swelling in the scrotum
- Those who are known to be immunocompromised and have significant signs or symptoms

SURGERY

Gynaecology
Spontaneous miscarriage flowchart

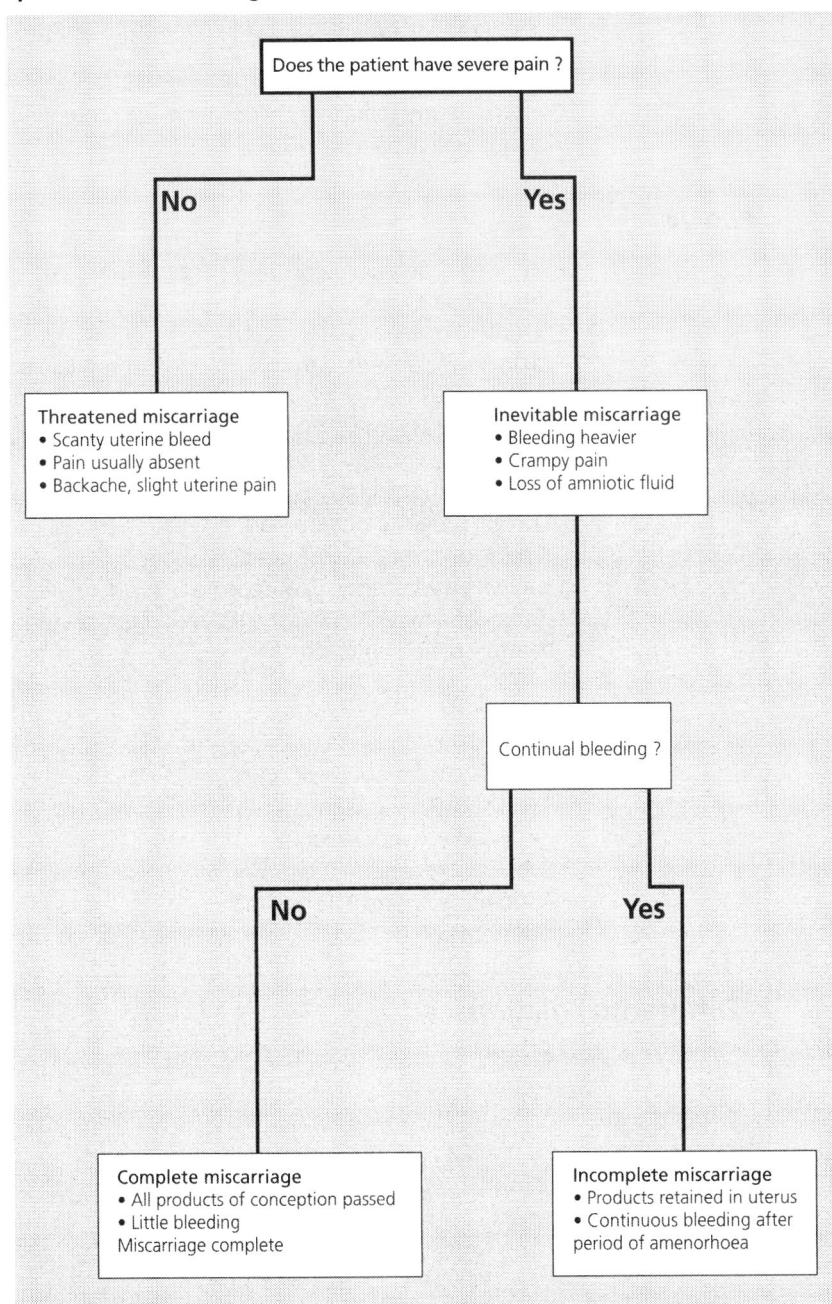

```
                    Does the patient have severe pain?
                    /                              \
                  No                              Yes
                  /                                \
Threatened miscarriage                    Inevitable miscarriage
• Scanty uterine bleed                    • Bleeding heavier
• Pain usually absent                     • Crampy pain
• Backache, slight uterine pain           • Loss of amniotic fluid

                                          Continual bleeding?
                                          /              \
                                        No              Yes
                                        /                \
                    Complete miscarriage              Incomplete miscarriage
                    • All products of conception       • Products retained in uterus
                      passed                           • Continuous bleeding after
                    • Little bleeding                    period of amenorhoea
                    Miscarriage complete
```

Ruptured ectopic pregnancy

Pregnancy outside the uterine cavity, usually occurs at 5–9 weeks of pregnancy, the commonest site being in the fallopian tube.

Consider in **any** female of childbearing age presenting with abdominal pain or collapse

What to ask

- Pain – constant, unilateral, may have referred shoulder pain
- History of ovarian cysts
- Factors which increase the risk of ectopic pregnancy include:
  - Previous gynaecological surgery
  - Pelvic inflammatory disease
  - Infertility treatment
  - Taking progesterone-only pill
  - Presence of intrauterine device
- Vaginal bleed, scanty, dark brown
- History of amenorrhoea last 4–8 weeks (may present before a period is missed!)

What to look for

An acute rupture will present with:
- Signs of shock – prolonged capillary refill, tachycardia, hypotension
- Sudden, severe pain
- Abdomen signs may be minimal
  Get help

Differential diagnoses
- Incomplete miscarriage
- Ovarian cyst with rupture/ torsion
- Appendicitis
- Pelvic inflammatory disease

SURGERY

Investigations

- FBC, U&E's, glucose, β-human chorionic gonadotrophin (β-hCG), cross match 6 units
- Rhesus and antibody status

Management

- Reassure the patient
- Two large-bore IV access cannulae and fluid resuscitation (patient may deteriorate at any time!)

Who to admit

Refer all patients to the on-call gynaecologist

ILLNESS

Bleeding in early pregnancy

Fetal loss before 24 weeks of pregnancy; 15–20% of women will miscarry in early pregnancy; for some this will not be their first miscarriage.

What to ask

- Known pregnancy and approximate dates
- Pain – some will have severe pain others a mild backache
- Any vaginal bleeding, quantity of bleed

What to look for

- Ask yourself is this a possible ectopic pregnancy
- Signs of shock: prolonged capillary refill, tachycardia, hypotension – if present **Get help**
- If abdominal tenderness or signs of peritonism, consider other possible diagnoses

Investigations

- FBC, U&E's, cross match, βhCG
- Rhesus factor

Management

- Reassure and explain what may be happening.
- Fluid resuscitation if signs of shock (two large IV cannulae)

Who to admit

- Discuss all cases with gynaecologist.
- Liaise as to who will give anti-D to rhesus-negative women. It must be given within 72 hours and not forgotten

SURGERY

Orthopaedics
Joint problems flowchart

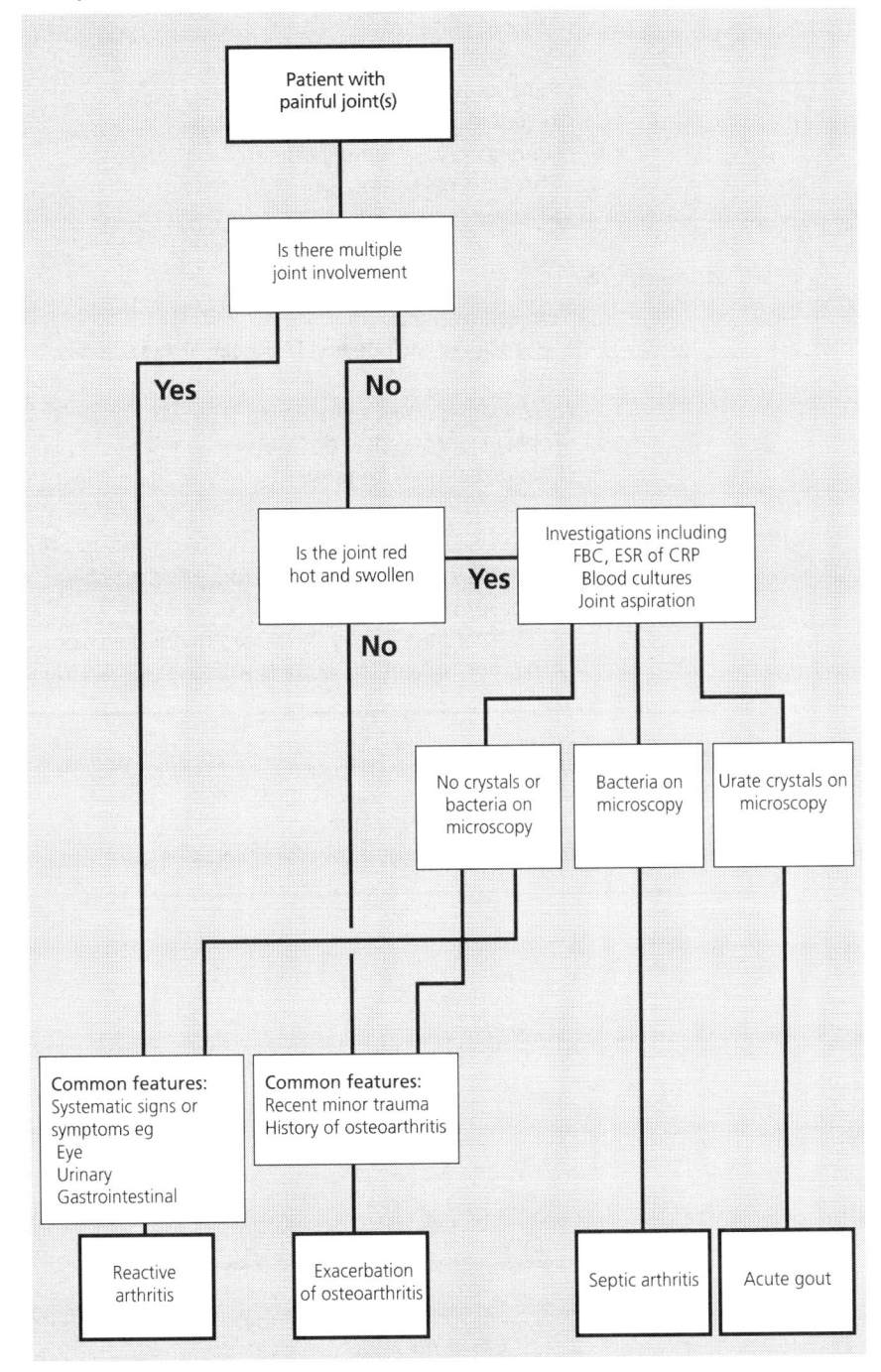

```
                    Patient with
                    painful joint(s)
                          │
                          ▼
                    Is there multiple
                    joint involvement
                    ┌─────┴─────┐
                  Yes           No
                   │             │
                   │             ▼
                   │       Is the joint red      Yes    Investigations including
                   │       hot and swollen ─────────►   FBC, ESR of CRP
                   │             │                      Blood cultures
                   │             No                     Joint aspiration
                   │             │                             │
                   │             │             ┌───────────────┼───────────────┐
                   │             │             ▼               ▼               ▼
                   │             │       No crystals or   Bacteria on     Urate crystals on
                   │             │       bacteria on      microscopy      microscopy
                   │             │       microscopy
                   │             │             │               │               │
         ┌─────────┘             │             │               │               │
         ▼                       ▼                             │               │
   Common features:        Common features:                    │               │
   Systematic signs or     Recent minor trauma                 │               │
   symptoms eg             History of osteoarthritis           │               │
   Eye                                                         │               │
   Urinary                                                     │               │
   Gastrointestinal                                            │               │
         │                       │                             │               │
         ▼                       ▼                             ▼               ▼
    Reactive              Exacerbation                    Septic arthritis   Acute gout
    arthritis             of osteoarthritis
```

Gout

What to ask

- Previous episodes
- Precipitating factors
- Dehydration
- Recent increased alcohol/protein intake
- Drug history – diuretics, aspirin
- Chronic renal failure
- Myeloproliferative disorders

What to look for

- Swollen red joint
- Typical joints include first MTPJ, tarsal joints, ankle, knee
- Excruciatingly painful to move
- Tophi in longstanding disease
- Mild pyrexia may be present

Investigations

- FBC, U&E's, glucose, urate – serum urate may be normal or high
- X-ray – chronically may show asymmetrical erosions
- Aspiration of joint will make the diagnosis definitively

Aspirating joints

- Get a senior to show you how
  Make sure you use an aseptic technique
  Send aspirate for microscopy – will show urate crystals in gout

SURGERY

Management

- Adequate analgesia including:
  - NSAIDs
  - Colchicine can be used if NSAIDs are contraindicated. Be careful as colchicine is contraindicated in patients with haematological, renal, and hepatic dysfunction
- Advise rest and elevation of the joint
- Advise the patient to see their GP if the attack doesn't settle within a week

ILLNESS

Septic arthritis

What to ask

- Duration of symptoms
- Any recent local penetrating trauma/surgery to joint
- Known joint problems, eg rheumatoid arthritis, joint replacement
- Any urethral/vaginal discharge (gonococcal arthritis)
- Drug history – steroids
- Immunocompromised patients

What to look for

- Red hot swollen joint
- Pyrexia
- Any movement of the joint is extremely painful
- Signs may be less apparent in the hip joint and elderly

Infections associated with septic arthritis

- **Gonorrhoea** – usually young man or woman with urethral/vaginal discharge
- **Lyme disease** – tick bite associated with spreading erythematous rash (erythema migrans)
- **Tuberculosis** – often hip/ knee and associated with night sweats and weight loss

Investigation

- FBC, U&E's, glucose, ESR or C-reactive protein, blood cultures
- Joint aspiration is essential in making the diagnosis in most cases – get someone to show you how
- X-rays – only if other diagnosis suspected or long-standing infection

Management

- Adequate analgesia
- If septic arthritis suspected or confirmed refer to orthopaedic doctor

SURGERY

Back pain

What to ask

- If there is a history of injury see Back injury (page 172–173)
- Previous back problems
- Alteration of bowel/bladder function
- Neurological symptoms
- Systemic symptoms, eg weight loss, night sweats
- Don't forget other causes of back pain:
  - Leaking abdominal aortic aneurysm (see page 89)
  - Acute pancreatitis (see page 92)
  - Renal/gynaecological disease

What to look for

- Systemic disturbance, eg pyrexia, anaemia
- Localised spinal tenderness
- Neurological examination including perineal sensation

Investigations

- X-rays of the lumbar spine are rarely useful and expose the patient to a high radiation dose
- Exceptions include:
  - Systemic symptoms or signs present
  - Exclusion of metastases from known malignancy
  - Children or elderly with severe/persistent pain
- If systemic features – FBC, ESR, blood cultures, etc.

Management

- All patients must be given adequate analgesia – if severe, IV morphine may be needed for pain/spasm

Who to refer

- Those with an alteration in bowel/bladder control or of perineal sensation indicating possible cauda equina syndrome
- Those with possible infection, malignancy/other systemic cause

continues overleaf

ILLNESS

- Those with new neurological signs
- Those unable to achieve satisfactory analgesia

If sending a patient home:
- Ensure they have adequate analgesia
- Advise gentle mobilisation and gradual return to normal activity
- Advise to return if bladder or bowel disturbance occurs

SURGERY

Joint problems – diagnosis uncertain

> Always exclude septic arthritis before making another diagnosis. This may require joint aspiration if the diagnosis is not obvious

Other causes of painful joints in the absence of trauma

Osteoarthritis
- A flare-up may occur without any remembered trauma to the joint
- Previous symptoms and effusion are normally present
- Treat with simple analgesia and rest but not immobility

Pseudogout
- Usually affects hip, wrist or knee in the elderly
- Calcification seen in joints on X-ray
- Treat in similar way to gout

Rarer conditions normally presenting with a polyarthritis

- Reiter's syndrome – associated with conjunctivitis, urethritis and arthritis
- Salmonella/shigella/campylobacter infection – may be complicated by an acute arthritis
- Rheumatic fever – mainly children 1–5 weeks after a streptococcal sore throat
- Acute onset of rheumatoid arthritis/juvenile chronic arthritis – very rare for initial presentation to be to the Emergency department
- Sickle cell crisis – may present with bone or joint pain (*see* page 74–75)
- Viral diseases – rubella, AIDS, hepatitis B

ILLNESS

Part B
INJURY

Assault	128
Major injury	130
Burns	132
Swallowed/inhaled foreign bodies	134
Minor wound care	136
Injury according to location	146

INJURY

INJURY

Assault

The following provides a few tips on treating the assaulted patient. Remember each assault is an alleged assault. Accurate and detailed documentation is essential, as at a later date it is likely you will be asked to provide a police statement. Use diagrams where possible.

The events

Most assaults are as a result of drunken fights. Remember domestic violence does occur and your patient may be reluctant to disclose any information due to fear of the repercussions. Ask for help from the senior nursing staff regarding your local policy for looking after these patients. Remember simply treating their wounds is not going to treat the underlying problem.

Alcohol

Many patients will be under the influence of alcohol. This can make the assessment difficult. X-rays may be inadequate as the patient may be unable to co-operate. If the patient is at risk bring them in overnight, otherwise arrange for them to return the next morning.

If your patient has decreased or fluctuating consciousness do not assume this is due to alcohol. **Get help**

Documentation and procedure

The patient may have lots of injuries, be methodical in your exam.
- Where, when, mechanism (glass bottle, hammer, baseball bat)
- Document all injuries – incision/laceration/bruising/abrasion. Remember the 5 Ss
- Symptoms following the assault – loss of consciousness/headache/vomiting/disturbance of

ASSAULT

vision or balance
- Perform the appropriate X-rays but do not be pressured into performing X-rays for legal reasons
- Document any treatments, eg steristrips/sutures
- Don't forget to ask about tetanus status and treat human bites (see page 143)
- Some departments have facilities to take photos for domestic violence patients
- Make sure your patient is going home with a responsible adult.

The 5 Ss
- **S**ite
- **S**ize (shape)
- **S**harp/blunt
- **S**terile – clean or contaminated
- **S**tructures – tendon/nerves/blood vessels and bones

The statement

- This is likely to come a few weeks later so your only aid is your documentation
- Get your first few checked. It is fact, not opinion that you are providing
- Finally don't forget to fill in your claim form!

INJURY

Major injury

Usually the ambulance service will inform you in advance of incoming major trauma, use this time to **Get help** as no one can deal with this by themselves.

What to ask

- **A**llergies
- **M**edications
- **P**ast medical history and pregnancy
- **L**ast ate at what time
- **E**vents leading up to the injury

What to look for

Perform a primary survey and treat any life-threatening injuries as you find them. Primary survey is:
- **A**IRWAY AND CERVICAL SPINE
- **B**REATHING
- **C**IRCULATION AND HAEMORRHAGE CONTROL

Investigations

- Do not delay immediate life-threatening treatments to perform investigations. The team leader will direct you to do specific investigations as required

Management

- The team leader will direct you to do a specific task, these could include:
  - **Airway and cervical spine** – give the patient 100% oxygen and if the airway is not open perform simple airway opening manoeuvres whilst maintaining in-line immobilisation of the c-spine
  - **Breathing** – look at the patient's chest and pattern of breathing to identify early on any serious chest injuries

MAJOR INJURY

- **Circulation and haemorrhage control** – ensure there are two large-bore cannulae and commence IV fluids rapidly and reassess. Apply direct pressure to any obvious external sources of bleeding

INJURY

Burns

If the patient has evidence of significant burns to the face, difficulty breathing or has had major trauma – **Get help**

What to ask

- Mechanism of injury especially what caused the burn, eg water, fire, hot fat, radiator, electricity or chemicals
- Associated injuries or effects of smoke inhalation
- First aid measures taken such as cold water
- Tetanus status (see page 144–145)

What to look for

- If evidence of burns around the mouth or respiratory signs then **Get help**
- Assess the depth:
  - **Superficial** – simple erythema
  - **Partial thickness** – superficial skin loss with some fluid exudate and pain
  - **Full thickness** – thick leathery areas with no sensation or capillary refill
- Assess the size to determine body surface area (BSA) involved, do not include erythema:
  - Palm of patient's hand including fingers is just under 1% of BSA
  - Use a Lund and Browder chart
  - Rule of nines: head 9%, each arm 9%, each leg 18%, front of trunk 18%, back of trunk 18%, perineum 1% (not applicable in children)

Management

- Adequate analgesia – may need IV morphine and tetanus (see page 144–145)

BURNS

- **Major burns**
  - >15% BSA in an adult **Get help** and commence IV fluids as local policy
  - >5% full thickness or involvement of face/head/neck/perineum/soles of feet/palms or circumferential burns discuss with senior or on-call plastic surgeon
- **Minor burns**
  - Use cold soaks and then dress with burns dressing as used in your department
  - Arrange follow-up according to departmental policy
- **Chemical and electrical burns**
  - Discuss with senior or on-call plastic surgeon

INJURY

Swallowed/inhaled foreign bodies

What to ask

- Swallowed or inhaled
- What was it
- When did it happen
- What symptoms does the patient have

What to look for

- **Signs of airway obstruction – Get help**. Gagging, drooling, vomiting, coughing, stridor, wheeze
- Rate and pattern of breathing, asymmetrical air entry
- Surgical emphysema in the neck
- Dysphagia, excess salivation suggestive of oesophageal impaction
- Check tonsilar fossa and base of tongue for fish bones.

> Most patients have swallowed the fish bone but it has scratched the oesophagus or pharynx causing discomfort

Investigations

- Perform X-rays based on signs and symptoms. Start with abdominal X-ray, if not seen move on to do chest X-ray and then cervical spine X-ray
- For a fish bone that is not seen on examination, do a soft tissue X-ray of the neck; look for the bone, and soft tissue swelling
- On chest X-ray look for: compensatory hyperinflation on an expiratory film, collapse, and consolidation.

> When X-rayed: a coin in the larynx appears side on as a bar, in the oesophagus as a round disc!

SWALLOWED/INHALED FOREIGN BODIES

Management

- If airway compromised, don't move the patient, **Get help** quickly
- Ensure airway patent
- Treat any emergency that arises because of the foreign body

---

If alkaline batteries or sharp object swallowed/inhaled discuss management with senior doctor

---

Who needs referral

Refer to on-call ENT doctor if:
- If patient has swallowed a fish bone and has complete dysphagia/bone seen on X-ray/severe or worsening symptoms or symptoms persisting beyond 24 hours
- If patient has inhaled a foreign body
- If patient has swallowed a foreign body and has airway compromise/oesophageal impaction/prevertebral soft tissue swelling or surgical emphysema
- If foreign body is below the diaphragm and patient is asympyomatic, send home and advise to return if GI symptoms develop

INJURY

Minor wound care

The following is a basic overview of how to examine and treat wounds. This largely depends on the location and severity of a wound and no two wounds will be identical, therefore if in doubt get help!

What to ask

- Mechanism of injury
- When did the injury occur
- Could there be glass or other foreign body in the wound
- Tetanus status, previous medical history: diabetic, on steroids or anticoagulants

What to look for

- Extent of soft tissue damage, and underlying structures
- Uncontrollable bleeding – apply pressure and **Get help**
- Dirty wound/evidence of infection
- Nerve damage (test before lignocaine infiltration)
- Tendon damage

Discuss with senior if:
- Stab wound
- Old wound (more than 12 h old)
- Infected wound
- Underlying tendon/nerve damage
- Wound very contaminated

MINOR WOUND CARE

Document the 5 Ss
- **S**ite
- **S**ize (shape)
- **S**harp/blunt
- **S**terile – clean or contaminated
- **S**tructures – tendon/nerves/blood vessels and bones

Investigation

- X-ray of appropriate area if looking for foreign body or fracture/dislocation (crush injuries likely to have fracture)

Management

Methods of closure include suture/steristrip/glue. If unsure discuss with senior.
- Ensure thorough examination for every wound going through the full thickness of the skin. Infiltrate with lignocaine if necessary
- Irrigate the wound thoroughly
- Close appropriately
- Ensure tetanus/ antibiotics given if indicated
- Advise on signs of infection and arrange appropriate follow-up.
- Refer patients with nerve and or tendon damage to the appropriate team.

Indications for antibiotics
- Open fracture
- Soft tissue infection
- Human or animal bite (*see* page 143)

INJURY

INJURY

Suturing a basic wound

After full examination and exclusion of a foreign body in a wound you may decide to close the wound with sutures. The following provides a few points to remember. Get somebody to show you how to suture.

The procedure

- Make sure your patient is comfortable, ideally lying down
- Explain the procedure
- Make sure they know they will have a scar and obtain their consent
- Infiltrate the area with local anaesthetic; for digits do a digital nerve block
- **Never** use local anaesthetic with epinephrine in fingers, toes, nose, ears or penis
- Clean thoroughly and explore wound
- Use the sutures preferred in your department. Plan the suturing: starting in the middle is usually the easiest and gives the best result
- Document the volume of lignocaine used and number of sutures required

Local anaesthetics

- **Lignocaine** – maximum dose is 3 mg/kg; 1% lignocaine = 10 mg/ml; anaesthesia lasts 30-60 min
- **Bupivacaine** – maximum dose is 2 mg/kg; 0.5% bupivocaine = 5 mg/ml anaesthesia lasts 3–8 hours

Suture size – these are the sizes usually used but are not a hard and fast rule

- Face 6/0, removal in 3–5 days
- Scalp, trunk 3/0, removal 7–10 days
- Limbs 4/0, removal 7–10 days
- Hands 4/0, removal in 7–10 days

MINOR WOUND CARE

Wounds that should be discussed before suturing

- Resulting from a crush injury, further swelling may lead to tissue necrosis; review 2–3 days later
- Dirty wounds, clean and debride, leave open and review in 2–3 days
- Bite wounds

INJURY

INJURY

Soft tissue infection

What to ask

- Duration
- Any wound or bite as possible source
- Feeling unwell or noticed a fever
- Pain
- Previous episodes
- Known diabetic or on steroids
- Athletes foot

What to look for

- Skin: erythema, swelling, warmth at the site
- Site and size of erythema
- Tracking of erythema (lymphangitis)
- Localised collection suggesting abscess
- If over a joint, consider septic arthritis
- Systemic signs – pyrexial, tachycardic

Investigations

- Capillary blood glucose
- FBC, U&E's, blood cultures if systemically unwell
- Demarcate area of erythema with indelible ink
- Swab if any pus or exudate

Management

> **My department's policy on antibiotics for soft tissue infection:**

Who needs referral

- If systemically unwell
- If not settling on oral antibiotics
- Diabetics/immunocompromised

MINOR WOUND CARE

If sending patient home

- Advise to rest and elevate affected limb
- Antibiotics
- Review in 2 days

Patient education!

Most patients are unaware of how serious this condition can be. They must have a low threshold for returning if it becomes worse despite treatment

INJURY

Needlestick injury

What to ask

- When and where did it occur
- Community-acquired or acquired at work as a healthcare provider
- Is the injured person immunised against hepatitis B
- Source of the needlestick injury and any known blood-borne diseases
- Tetanus status

Management

Injured person
- Encourage wound to bleed and wash thoroughly with soap and water
- Take 10 ml of clotted blood for baseline storage
- If injured person has never been immunised against hepatitis B, discuss with your senior regarding your department's policy
- Give tetanus if needed

Source
- If possible take a 10-ml sample of clotted blood. The injured person must not ask for consent or take the blood, but delegate the task to someone else; consent for testing for infectivity must be obtained
- If the source is suspected HIV positive, you cannot test for HIV without consent; get help regarding further management for the injured person

> Reassure the injured person that the risk of HIV infection from a needlestick injury or human bite is very low, but that if they are concerned they can have counselling and be offered an HIV test 3 months later

MINOR WOUND CARE

Bites

What to ask

- Type of bite (insect, human, animal)
- Time of bite
- Onset and type of symptoms
- Tetanus status

What to look for

- Erythema
- Swelling
- Tenderness
- Infection
- Systemic effects: difficulty breathing, signs of shock/ signs of allergic reaction
- Consider possibility of retained tooth

Management

- Clean wound thoroughly
- Insect bite
  - Antihistamine for local reaction
  - Consider antibiotics for infection
- Animal bite
  - Discuss with a senior regarding closure
  - Antibiotics if skin penetrated
  - Tetanus
- Human bite
  - Antibiotics
  - Tetanus
  - Hepatitis B prophylaxis/consider the risk of HIV, see Needlestick injury (page 142)

My department's policy on antibiotics for bites:

Who to admit

- For those with a severe infection as a result of the bite, consider IV antibiotics. See Soft tissue infection (page 140–141)

INJURY

Tetanus immunisation

Divide wounds into *tetanus-prone* and *non-tetanus-prone/clean* wounds.

Tetanus-prone wounds include those which:
- Are more than 6 hours old at presentation
- Are stab/puncture-type wounds
- Contain devitalised tissue
- Are contaminated with soil/manure
- Are clinically infected

Due to the rising incidence of diphtheria, all adults needing a booster should have a tetanus-diphtheria booster (**Td**).

Tetanus immunoglobulin dose is 250 IU – give 500 IU if the wound is over 24 hours old or the patient weighs over 90 kg.

Routine tetanus immunisation in the UK began in 1961. Individuals born before then may not have been immunised. Most people in the armed forces have had a full course

MINOR WOUND CARE

Immunisation status	Clean wound	Tetanus-prone wound
Five doses of tetanus toxoid in lifetime (course + two boosters)	Nil	Consider tetanus immunoglobulin if particularly high risk, eg manure contamination
Complete course or booster within last 10 years (fewer than 5 doses in lifetime)	Nil	Consider tetanus immunoglobulin if particularly high risk, eg manure contamination
Complete course or booster over 10 years ago (fewer than 5 doses in lifetime)	Tetanus toxoid booster (Td)	Tetanus toxoid booster (Td) and tetanus immunoglobulin
Not immunised	Tetanus toxoid course	Tetanus toxoid course and tetanus immunoglobulin
Tetanus status unknown	Patient to check with GP within 72 hours – may need booster/course/ antibody level check	Tetanus immunoglobulin and patient to check with GP within 72 hours – may need booster or course

INJURY

Injury according to location
Head

What to ask

- Mechanism of injury. Beware of the large force over a small surface area, eg golf club
- Witnessed loss of consciousness
- Nausea or frequency of vomiting
- Disturbance of vision or balance
- Headache unrelieved by painkillers
- Amnesia pre and/or post event
- Any fitting
- On anticoagulants

> Always consider the possibility of a C-spine injury in any head injury

What to look for

- Assess GCS if less than 12 **Get help**
- Local tenderness, swelling and bruising
- Neurological signs: test cranial nerves, check eye movements and pupils
- Signs of basal skull fracture: bilateral peri-orbital haematoma/bruising around the mastoid area/blood in the auditory meatus and behind the eardrum
- Palpate any open wound for fracture

Investigations

My department's policy on radiological investigations:

INJURY ACCORDING TO LOCATION

Who needs referral

Admit patients
- Taking oral anticoagulants or who have a bleeding disorder
- GCS is <15
- No responsible adult to watch them
- Had a fit
- Has significant degree of amnesia

If safe to be discharged ensure the patient goes home with a responsible adult who will supervise them overnight.

Head injury advice for the patient going home:
- It is common to have post-concussion symptoms – headache, dizziness, poor memory and concentration, tiredness and irritability. If these are still present after 2 weeks, see your GP
- Avoid alcohol, television, computer games, sleeping medication and contact sport
- Return if experiencing persistent vomiting, severe headache, or loss of coordination
- Take regular analgesia

INJURY

Face

What to ask

- Mechanism of injury – vast majority will be assaults
- Alteration of vision – record visual acuity
- Altered sensation to face
- Dental injury (see page 150–151)
- Head injury symptoms (see page 146–147)

What to look for

- Swelling, tenderness and wounds – document well as these patients often end up needing a Police statement
- Neurological deficit – altered sensation over cheek and lip signifies infraorbital nerve injury and usually a fracture
- Subconjunctival haemorrhage – if unable to identify posterior margin usually associated with orbital fracture
- Head injury signs (see page 146–147)

Investigation

- Facial X-rays – notoriously difficult to interpret; look for:
  - Symmetry
  - Maxillary sinuses should be clear – fluid levels or opacity usually indicate fracture
  - The zygomatic complex has four attachments – look for steps or displacement in each:
    superiorly to the frontal bone
    inferiorly to the wall of the maxillary sinus
    medially to the infraorbital margin
    laterally across the arch to the temporal bone
- Mandibular X-rays – check both sides as the mandible usually fractures in two places

Management

- Facial wounds – majority can be closed with glue or steristrips. If sutures are required be sure you have

INJURY ACCORDING TO LOCATION

the skills to do a good job, in particular with eyebrows and the vermilion border of the lip, which if not done accurately can leave a disfiguring scar for life
- Facial fracture – discuss with senior or maxillo-facial surgeon

Nose injuries

X-rays are not helpful. Always check for:
- Septal haematoma (red swelling on septum) – if seen refer to ENT doctor
- Nasal deformity or septal deviation – arrange for ENT clinic follow-up either immediately or if noticed by patient once the swelling has settled

INJURY

Dental complaints

What to ask

- Get a clear mechanism of injury to identify what structures could be involved, think about facial injuries (see page 148–149)
- If a tooth has been avulsed ask how the tooth has been stored since the injury
- Head injury symptoms (see page 146–147)

What to look for

- Swelling, tenderness and wounds – document well as if assaulted these patients often end up needing a police statement
- Head injury signs (see page 146–147)
- If avulsed tooth look for damage to the socket that may need surgical repair
- Inability to fully open the mouth or bite down on closed mouth can suggest mandibular injury

Investigation

- X-rays are not necessary unless you suspect a mandibular injury
- If an avulsed tooth or part of a tooth cannot be accounted for then consider aspiration and request a chest X-ray

Management

- Simple chipped teeth can be referred back to dentist
- Avulsed teeth need reimplantation by maxillo-facial surgeon unless child's milk tooth – if possible replace tooth temporarily in the socket and ask patient to hold it there
- Mandibular fracture – discuss with senior or maxillo-facial surgeon

INJURY ACCORDING TO LOCATION

Dental abscess
This commonly presents at night, prescribe analgesia, eg ibuprofen 400 mg tds and antibiotic. Refer to dentist.

My department's policy for antibiotics in dental abscess:

Eye

What to ask

- Mechanism of injury
- If high velocity (eg using hammer and chisel) consider intra-ocular foreign body
- If blunt or penetrating injury
  If there is a penetrating injury to the eye **Get help immediately**

Visual acuity

The visual acuity is recorded as:
the distance the patient is from the chart (usually 6 m)/the number next to the line of text the patient can see, eg 6/18

Problems

- If the patient has forgotten their glasses then use a pinhole
- If the patient can't see any of the letters then use finger counting

What to look for

- If the patient is unable to keep their eye open for examination – use local anaesthetic drops
- Visual acuity – must be recorded in **all** patients
- Use fluorescein drops and look for uptake (shows green with a blue light indicating damage to the epithelium)
- Check for:
  - Foreign bodies (FBs)
  - Abrasions – show as fluorescein uptake
  - Hyphaema – blood in anterior chamber – may look hazy or as a horizontal level
- Always evert the eyelid (get someone to show you how) to look for subtarsal FBs

Management

- If a FB is seen, use a local anaesthetic and remove – get someone to show you how
- After removing a metallic FB a 'rust ring' may remain – ask about your department's policy for removal of this
- If you suspect an intra-ocular FB (high-velocity mechanism and no FB is seen on cornea) discuss with a senior or ophthalmologist
- If an abrasion is seen treat with antibiotic ointment – healing normally occurs within 1–2 days. Large abrasions may need review
- If hyphaema is seen or there is altered vision after a blunt injury, refer to an ophthalmologist

Neck

> If any of the following are present:
> - High-impact RTA or other dangerous mechanism of injury
> - Persisting neurological symptoms
> - Neurological signs
> - Known to have ankylosing spondylitis or rheumatoid arthritis
>
> Immobilise the neck immediately – lie the patient down, hold the head in a neutral position and get help to apply head blocks and tape

What to ask

- Mechanism of injury in detail, ie height of fall, if RTA – vehicles and speeds involved, seat belts/airbags
- Immediate or delayed onset of neck pain
- Neurological symptoms

What to look for

- Cervical spine tenderness
- Neurological signs

Investigations

- Use the Canadian cervical spine rule to decide whether to X-ray (see page 156)

INJURY ACCORDING TO LOCATION

X-ray interpretation

- Take your time with cervical spine X-rays and if you are unsure get a second opinion

A system for looking at cervical spine X-rays

A – is the X-ray **A**dequate (C1–C7/T1 junction) and are the vertebrae **A**ligned
? – are the curves of the spine smooth and is the odontoid peg in the correct position – get someone to show you this
B – trace round the **B**ones and check for any steps or cortical breaks
C – look at the **C**artilages and joints checking for alignment and equal intervertebral disc space height
S – check there is no bulging of the **S**oft tissue stripe anterior to the vertebral bodies

Management

- If you see or suspect a fracture – **Get help**
- For whiplash-type injuries:
   - Encourage movement of the neck
   - Regular analgesia – NSAIDs if possible
   - Local warmth, eg hot towel eases stiffness
   - Physiotherapy according to local guidelines
   - Warn that recovery may take several weeks

INJURY

Neck

Canadian cervical spine rule flowchart

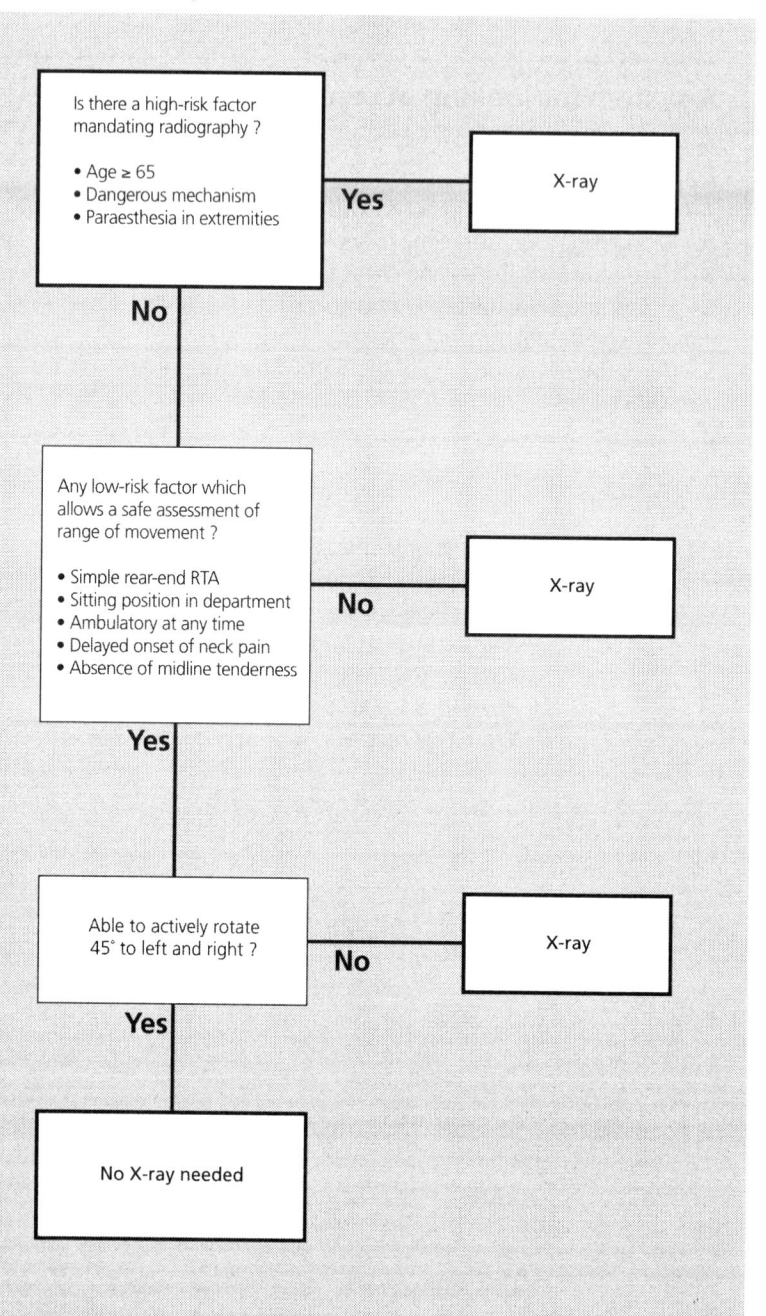

```
Is there a high-risk factor
mandating radiography?

• Age ≥ 65
• Dangerous mechanism          ──Yes──▶  X-ray
• Paraesthesia in extremities

         │ No
         ▼

Any low-risk factor which
allows a safe assessment of
range of movement?

• Simple rear-end RTA
• Sitting position in department  ──No──▶  X-ray
• Ambulatory at any time
• Delayed onset of neck pain
• Absence of midline tenderness

         │ Yes
         ▼

Able to actively rotate
45° to left and right?  ──No──▶  X-ray

         │ Yes
         ▼

No X-ray needed
```

INJURY ACCORDING TO LOCATION

When to X-ray

• Use the Canadian C-Spine Rule

Dangerous mechanisms include:

• Fall from elevation greater than 1 metre or five stairs
• Axial load to head
• High-speed RTA > 60 mph or rollover/ejection
• Off-road RTA
• Bicycle collision

Simple rear-end collision excludes:

• Pushed into oncoming traffic
• Hit by bus or truck
• Rollover
• Hit by high-speed vehicle

INJURY

Chest

What to ask

If potential penetrating injury or major trauma – **Get help**
- Mechanism of injury
- Time of injury
- Character, site and onset of pain
- Pain worse on movement or deep breathing
- Breathlessness, haemoptysis
- If there was no injury you must consider cardiac/pulmonary causes for the pain

What to look for

- Equal air entry and percussion bilaterally
- Observe chest wall movements for possible flail segment

Flail segment

The chest moves paradoxically inwards during inspiration and outwards during expiration. Caused by a fracture of three or more ribs in two places. Indicates association with damage to underlying lung

---

- Document the oxygen saturation and respiratory rate; if abnormal could be suggestive of pneumothorax
- If lower chest injury, suspect underlying abdominal organ injury
- If signs of shock: prolonged capillary refill time, hypotension etc – **Get help**

Investigations

- Chest X-ray if possible internal injury or multiple fractures; otherwise a rib fracture is a clinical diagnosis
- Sternal views
- ECG if suspected cardiac contusion; ECG may show signs of ischaemia, infarction or arrhythmia

INJURY ACCORDING TO LOCATION

Management

- Oxygen
- Adequate analgesia

Who to refer

- Elderly – if unable to cope at home
- Multiple rib fractures/flail segment
- Chronic co-existing lung disease
- Cardiac contusion
- Pneumothorax
- Chest infection
- Pain uncontrolled by adequate analgesia

Sending the patient home

- Advise the patient that the pain will initially become worse before it improves
- Advise regular simple pain relief, eg ibuprofen and paracetamol
- Explain the importance of good pain relief in order to breathe and cough as normal and thereby prevent chest infection (particularly in smokers)
- To return if any new symptoms develop, eg shortness of breath

INJURY

Shoulder

What to ask

- Mechanism of injury – usually falls
- Epileptic fit or direct blow to the shoulder – consider posterior dislocation
- Handedness and occupation
- Don't forget shoulder pain can be due to neck problems and diaphragmatic irritation

What to look for

- Bony tenderness over the clavicle, scapula, acromioclavicular joint and humeral head and neck
- A rounded contour – the deltoid looks squared off in anterior dislocation
- If no obvious fracture or dislocation, check abduction can be initiated – if not, consider a rotator cuff rupture
- Neurological examination and check for pulses if neurological symptoms or significant deformity

Investigations

- X-ray if bony tenderness or deformity. Check if acromioclavicular joint aligned and appearance of humeral head – if symmetrical (light bulb sign) consider posterior dislocation

Management

- Clavicle fracture – broad arm sling. Refer to orthopaedic doctor if overlying skin is tented/white
- Humeral head/neck fracture
  - Undisplaced fracture – broad arm sling.
  - Displaced or angulated fracture – discuss with a senior or orthopaedic doctor
- Dislocated shoulder
  - Anterior dislocation – get help to reduce this
  - Posterior dislocation – difficult to spot. Full external rotation is impossible. If suspected speak to a senior or orthopaedic doctor

INJURY ACCORDING TO LOCATION

- Acromioclavicular joint injury
  - Tender but no step on X-ray – broad arm sling
  - Step/separation on X-ray – discuss with senior or orthopaedic doctor
- Rotator cuff rupture – refer to orthopaedic doctor
- Soft tissue injury – adequate analgesia. Advise rest with early mobilisation. Follow-up if significant pain or reduction in movement according to departmental policy

Elbow

What to ask

- Handedness and job
- Mechanism of injury, eg fall onto outstretched hand (FOOSH)

What to look for

- Swelling/effusion
- Red/hot joint
- Bony tenderness to olecranon, epicondyles and radial head
- Neurovascular deficit, if any deficit refer to on-call orthopaedic doctor.
- Range of movement – supination, pronation, flexion, extension

> Full range of movement usually excludes any serious injury

- Dislocation

Investigations

- X-ray the elbow; if no fracture seen, look for fat pads

Management

- Appropriate analgesia
- Radial head fracture
  - Undisplaced – treat with collar and cuff and fracture clinic follow-up
  - Displaced or communited – discuss with on-call orthopaedic doctor
- Radial and ulnar shaft – refer both of the following to on-call orthopaedic doctor:
  - Monteggia fracture (distal ulna with dislocation of radial head)

INJURY ACCORDING TO LOCATION

- Galeazzi fracture (proximal radius and dislocation of inferior radio-ulnar joint at wrist)
- Olecranon fracture – displacement/anterior dislocation, discuss with on-call orthopaedic doctor
- Medial and lateral epicondyle fracture – check median and ulnar nerve. Refer to on-call orthopaedic doctor
- Elbow dislocation – loss of triangular relationship between olecranon and epicondyles. Check for median/ulnar nerve damage and brachial artery damage. Refer to on-call orthopaedic doctor
- Olecranon bursitis – inflammation/ swelling and pain. Make sure not a septic joint. *See* joint infections (page 122). Broad arm sling. Review as per local policy

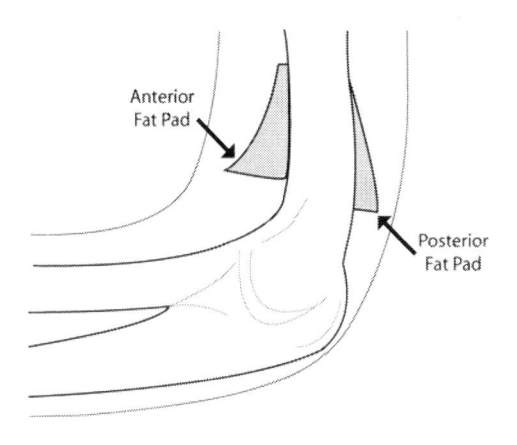

Anterior Fat Pad

Posterior Fat Pad

INJURY

INJURY

Forearm

What to ask

- Handedness and job
- Mechanism of injury, eg fall onto out stretched hand (FOOSH)
- Previous injuries
- *See* sections on elbow injuries (page 162–163) and wrist injuries (page 166–167)

What to look for

- Tenderness over radius or ulna, swelling or deformity
- Decreased range of movement or pain on particular movements, always remember supination and pronation
- Distal neurovascular deficit including radial pulse, if any deficit then refer to on-call orthopaedic doctor urgently

Investigations

- Request forearm X-rays but ensure you state where the patient is tender to allow radiographer to centre X-ray
- Remember that the two forearm bones form a ring and if you see a break look for a second break or dislocation in the other bone (study the wrist and elbow joints)

Management

- Appropriate analgesia
- Solitary undisplaced fractures of radius or ulna can be treated in above-elbow back slab (to stop supination) and fracture clinic follow-up
- All other fractures should be discussed with senior or on-call orthopaedic doctor

Compartment syndrome

- This can occur in any part of any limb. Essentially it is a build-up of pressure in a closed compartment, eg forearm. It occurs following the fracture of a long bone or there may be no history of injury, eg lying on arm for a length of time
- Loss of distal neurovascular function is a late sign and the diagnosis is made on the finding of severe pain out of proportion to findings and a high index of suspicion
- If suspected refer to on-call orthopaedic doctor

INJURY

Wrist

What to ask

- Handedness and job
- Mechanism of injury, eg fall onto out stretched hand (FOOSH)
- Previous injuries
- If no history of injury, ask about repetitive movements, eg typing or gardening
- See sections on hand (page 168–169) and forearm injuries (page 164–165)

What to look for

- Tenderness over radius, ulna, scaphoid and carpal bones
- Swelling or deformity (dinnerfork deformity in Colles' fracture)
- Decreased range of movement or pain on particular movements such as 'telescoping the thumb' in scaphoid injuries
- Distal neurovascular deficit including radial pulse, if any deficit then refer to on-call orthopaedic doctor urgently
- Consider scaphoid views

Scaphoid examination

- Tenderness in snuffbox
- Pain on ulnar deviation
- Pain on compression/telescoping of the thumb
- Tender over scaphoid tubercle

Investigations

- If distal radius or ulna fracture suspected get wrist views. If possible scaphoid fracture request scaphoid views (if local policy)
- As well as looking for bony injury, check on lateral view for alignment of capitate on lunate on distal radius

Management

- Appropriate analgesia (see page xi–xii)
- Undisplaced fractures of distal radius not involving joint surface – below elbow backslab and fracture clinic follow-up
- Colles' fracture – distal radius fragment angulated dorsally, discuss with senior or orthopaedics regarding manipulation
- Smith's fracture – distal radius angulated volarly (reverse of Colles' fracture), refer to on-call orthopaedic doctor
- All other wrist fractures should be discussed with senior or on-call orthopaedic doctor
- If tender over extensor aspect of wrist with or without crepitus and no fracture, consider tenosynovitis. Treat with NSAIDs, immobilisation and review according to local policy

INJURY

Hand

Hands are a major source of litigation. Document everything you have examined: if it is not documented, you have not done it! Remove any rings immediately

What to ask

- What happened and when
- Handedness and job

What to look for

- Injury to: skin, nails, bones, joints, tendons, ligaments, nerves and vessels
- Deformity, dislocation, swelling
- Bony tenderness and range of movement of joints
- Test flexor profundus: flexion at DIPJ with other joints fixed (allows power grip)
- Test flexor digitorum superficialis: flexion at MCPJ with all other fingers extended (allows fine movements)
- Test flexor pollicis longus (FPL): active flexion of IPJ of thumb
- Nerves: test sensation. Radial – dorsum hand, web space between thumb and index finger; ulna – little finger; median – index finger
- Look for ligament laxity specifically ulnar collateral ligament of the thumb. Usually caused by hyper-extension. Get someone to show you how to do this

---

- Compare both hands
- Name, do not number, digits
- Always examine wrist and forearm with a hand injury

Investigations

- X-ray appropriate view. Lateral and AP for the fingers. Oblique and AP for the hand
- Always X-ray crush injuries

Management

Get someone to show you how to do these procedures

INJURY ACCORDING TO LOCATION

Soft tissue
- Paronychia – digital nerve block, incise and drain, dressing
- Subungal haematomas – trephine the nail
- Laceration to nailbed – get somebody to show you how to repair this
- Finger tip injury – exclude bony injury and discuss management with a senior
- Crush injury – check for bony injury. Clean wound, avoid closure, elevate, pain relief and review

Tendon
- Tendon injuries refer to on-call orthopaedic/plastic surgeon
- Tendon sheath infections can result from small puncture wounds. Severe pain on passive extension, tenderness over the flexor tendon and swelling of the finger. Refer to orthopaedics
- Mallet finger – inability to fully actively extend DIPJ; if fracture >30% joint surface, refer to fracture clinic. Otherwise zimmer or mallet splint, follow-up in 6 wks

Bony injury
- Fifth metacarpal head/neck – typical punching injury. Neighbour strap, wool and crepe, follow-up. Look for tooth wound (*see* bites page 143)
- Base of first metacarpal (Bennett's) – refer to orthopaedics
- Look for rotational deformity with fractures of the hand. Refer to orthopaedics

Dislocations

Always X-ray before and after reduction
- Interphalangeal – Analgesia; reduction; neighbour strap; follow-up fracture clinic
- All other disclocations should be discussed with orthopaedic on-call

Pitfalls

- Does the patient need tetanus or antibiotics
- High-pressure injection injuries – can cause tracking of inflammatory agents and adhesions of tendons. Debridement may be necessary. Refer to orthopaedic or plastic surgeon

INJURY

Abdomen

If the patient has had major trauma **Get help** (see page 130–131)

What to ask

- Mechanism of injury, eg RTA, or direct blow
- Pre-existing abdominal disease

What to look for

- Signs of shock: tachycardia, prolonged capillary refill or hypotensive – **Get help**
- Localised or diffuse involuntary guarding and rebound tenderness
- Bruising to abdomen, eg from seatbelt

Investigations

- FBC, U&E's, blood glucose, LFTs, amylase, group and save
- Urinalysis
- Further investigations are best done after discussion with senior or surgical on-call team

Who needs referral

- If significant mechanism of injury or any abdominal signs then refer to on-call surgeons for assessment; titrate IV morphine/diamorphine for analgesia (see page xi–xii) and give an antiemetic

If sending the patient home

- Ensure someone responsible will be with them
- Tell them to return if symptoms change, worsen or persist, explaining potential for deterioration
- Ensure adequate analgesia

INJURY ACCORDING TO LOCATION

Pregnancy and abdominal injury

In pregnancy the uterus protects the other visceral organs but always look for injury to this organ suggested by:
- Uterine tenderness or easily palpable fetal parts
- Absence of fetal movements
- No fetal heart rate with Doppler ultrasound

Enquire about rhesus status. Refer to on-call obstetrician if uterine injury suspected

INJURY

INJURY

Back

What to ask

- Mechanism of injury – falls, RTAs are common causes
- Often associated with major trauma therefore ensure no other serious injuries are present – see major trauma (page 130–131)
- Pre-existing morbidity, eg osteoporosis, ankylosing spondylitis
- If minor trauma associated with longstanding back pain – see back pain (page 123–124)

If any of the following are present, immobilise the patient immediately by lying them down on a trolley and **get help**:
- Any neurological symptoms
- Neurological signs
- Any alteration in bowel or bladder control

What to look for

- If the patient is immobilised – log roll them to examine the back – you will need four other people to help you to do this
- Localised spinal tenderness/swelling
- Neurological assessment – including tone, power, reflexes, sensation

Investigation

- X-rays if bony tenderness or any neurological signs or symptoms
- Wedge fractures are often seen in elderly and it can be difficult to assess whether they are new or old – if in doubt get a senior or orthopaedic opinion

INJURY ACCORDING TO LOCATION

Management

- Only allow immobilisation to be removed if:
  - X-rays show no fracture **and**
  - There is no neurological deficit

Who needs referral

- Any fracture
- Persisting neurological symptoms
- Any new neurological sign

If sending the patient home

- Give adequate analgesia – advise patient to continue gentle activity and gradually return to normal activity

Pelvis, hip and thigh

If the patient has had major trauma – **Get help**

What to ask

- Mechanism of injury, eg RTA or fall from height
- Co-existing injuries especially in the elderly
- Was it a fall or a collapse (see page 33)

What to look for

- Signs of shock: tachycardia, prolonged capillary refill or hypotensive – **Get help**
- Associated abdominal injury (see page 170–171)
- Blood at the external meatus suggesting urethral damage
- Leg shortening or external rotation suggesting fractured neck of femur, check for neurovascular deficit
- Swelling or deformity in fractured femur

Investigations

- X-ray femur – hip to knee
- Pelvic X-ray or hip X-ray including lateral for neck of femur injuries
- Don't forget the pelvis is made up of three rings of bone, it is unusual to have only one injury
- Check Shenton's line or trabeculae disruption if possible fractured neck of femur

Management

- Adequate analgesia
- In femoral shaft fractures:
  - Arrange for splintage of the limb
  - Femoral block – get someone to show how to do this

INJURY ACCORDING TO LOCATION

Who needs referral

- Refer pubic rami fractures to on-call orthopaedic doctor or physicians depending on local policy
- Refer fracture shaft and/or neck of femur to on-call orthopaedic doctor and titrate IV morphine/diamorphine for analgesia (see page xi–xii) and give an antiemetic

> Beware in the elderly a normal hip X-ray does not exclude fracture. If appropriate mechanism of injury and inability to weight bear with normal X-ray then discuss with senior or orthopaedic doctor

INJURY

Knee

What to ask

- Mechanism of injury
  - Twisting often injures menisci
  - Valgus or varus strain = medial or lateral collateral ligament injury
  - Blow to medial aspect may dislocate patella
  - Penetrating injury may enter knee joint
- If swelling – how long it took to develop
  - Haemarthrosis within 2 hours
  - Effusion usually develops overnight
- If knee locked – stuck in flexion and unable to straighten

What to look for

- Effusion/haemarthrosis – either patellar tap or palpable fluid
- Swelling in front of the knee joint – prepatellar fluid
- Bony tenderness over the patella, tibial plateau and femoral condyles
- Joint line tenderness – suggests meniscal injury
- Dislocation of patella – knee is normally held in flexion
- Straight leg raising – implies intact extensor mechanism
- Stress the medial and lateral collateral ligaments with the knee in 20° flexion for pain and laxity
- Cruciate ligament rupture – positive anterior or posterior drawer sign

Investigations

- X-ray according to Ottawa knee rules
- On X-ray – check equal height of tibial plateau as plateau fractures can be difficult to identify

INJURY ACCORDING TO LOCATION

Ottawa knee rules

A knee X-ray is only required for acute knee injury patients with one or more of these findings:
- Aged 55 years or older **or**
- Tenderness at head of fibula **or**
- Isolated tenderness of patella **or**
- Inability to flex to 90° **or**
- Inability to weight bear both immediately and in the emergency department (four steps)

Management

- Dislocated patella – no X-ray is necessary – reduce by straightening leg with pressure over lateral side of patella. Treat with plaster cylinder
- Soft tissue injuries, meniscal injuries and collateral ligament sprains – **R**est, **I**ce packs, **C**ompression and **E**levation. Advise patient to exercise quadriceps muscle by straight leg raising for 10 seconds four times a day. Follow-up according to departmental policy
- Pre-patellar swellings
  - If associated with wound consider infection – discuss with senior or orthopaedic doctor
  - If no wound usually inflammatory – treat with NSAIDs, rest and ice packs

Who needs referral

- All fractures
- Cruciate ligament rupture
- Locked knee
- Quadriceps muscle rupture – indicated by inability to perform straight leg raise and gap in tendon on palpation
- Complete rupture of collateral ligament – stressing ligament produces significant joint movement
- Haemarthrosis – aspirate joint if no fracture seen (get someone to show you how); check cruciate ligaments

INJURY

Lower leg

What to ask

- Mechanism of injury
  - Sudden severe pain in calf or heel typical of Achilles or gastrocnemius tear
- Pre-tibial injury – if taking steroids or anticoagulants

What to look for

- Swelling, tenderness and deformity of tibial fracture
  - If wound – consider open fracture
  - Check neurovascular status
- Tenderness over gastrocnemius or Achilles
- Check Achilles continuity by feeling for gap in tendon and with Simmond's test:
  - Ask patient to kneel on a chair
  - Squeeze both calves in turn and check for equal plantar flexion of feet
  - Unequal plantar flexion indicates Achilles tear

Investigation

- X-rays of tibia and fibula if possible fracture
  - Check from knee to ankle
  - Tibia and fibula form a 'ring of bone' – a displaced fracture of one must be accompanied by another fracture or major ligamentous injury

Management

- Adequate analgesia and antibiotics if open fracture
- Gastrocnemius injury – early physiotherapy and follow-up according to departmental policy
- Pre-tibial injury – closure should be attempted with Steristrips if possible. If unable to close discuss with senior or plastic surgeon. Follow-up according to departmental policy

INJURY ACCORDING TO LOCATION

My hospital's antibiotic policy for open fracture is:

Who needs referral

- All tibial and fibular fractures
- Achilles tendon rupture – discuss with senior or orthopaedic doctor

INJURY

180 INJURY

Ankle

What to ask

- Mechanism of injury – inversion or eversion
- Ability to weight bear – initially and currently

What to look for

- Bony tenderness – malleoli, navicular, fifth metatarsal base and calcaneus
- Check Achilles tendon is intact and non-tender
- Neurological assessment and pulse check if neurological symptoms or significant deformity – **Get help**

Investigations

- Use Ottawa ankle rules to decide whether to X-ray
- Check if talar shift (joint space between talus and malleoli is wider on one side)

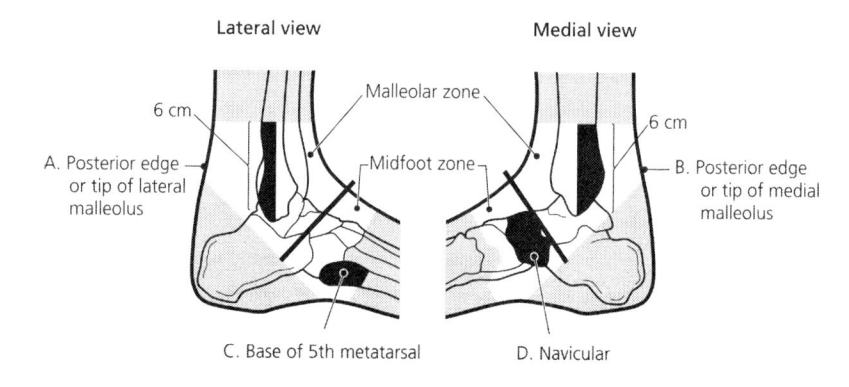

Lateral view

Medial view

6 cm

Malleolar zone

6 cm

A. Posterior edge or tip of lateral malleolus

Midfoot zone

B. Posterior edge or tip of medial malleolus

C. Base of 5th metatarsal

D. Navicular

An ankle X-ray series is required only if there is any pain in malleolar zone and any of these findings:	A foot X-ray series is required only if there is any pain in midfoot zone and any of these findings:
• Bone tenderness at A • Bone tenderness at B • Inability to bear weight both immediately and in emergency department	• Bone tenderness at C • Bone tenderness at D • Inability to bear weight both immediately and in emergency department

INJURY ACCORDING TO LOCATION

Management

- Soft tissue injury – RICE (**R**est, **I**ce packs, **C**ompression bandage and **E**levation). Crutches if unable to weight bear but encourage patient to mobilise as soon as possible. Arrange follow-up if significant pain or swelling
- Ankle fracture – discuss all fractures other than flake fractures with senior or orthopaedic doctor. Treat flake fractures with below-knee backslab
- Calcaneal and fifth metatarsal fracture – *see* foot injury (page 182–183)
- Achilles tendon injury – *see* lower leg injury (page 178–179)

INJURY

Foot

What to ask

- Mechanism of injury in particular:
  - Fall from height – consider calcaneus/talus injury (also examine hips, back and neck)
  - Associated with ankle injury – fifth metatarsal base and navicular fractures common
  - Repetitive strain, eg road running, consider stress fractures of metatarsal
- Ability to weight bear
- If crushed – approximate weight and time involved

What to look for

- Bony tenderness in ankle injures
  - over the base of the fifth metatarsal and navicular
- Calcaneal tenderness and bruising
- Neurovascular status in crush injuries

Investigations

- Calcaneal views should be asked for with suspected calcaneal injury
- Stress fractures do not normally become evident on X-ray until at least 2 weeks after the initial injury
- Second to fifth toes are not normally X-rayed unless possibly compound injury or obvious deformity

Management

- Calcaneal fractures – discuss with senior or orthopaedic doctor
- Fracture of the fifth metatarsal base – below-knee backslab and crutches
- Fracture of the navicular – below-knee backslab and crutches

INJURY ACCORDING TO LOCATION

- Metatarsal fracture – discuss with senior or orthopaedic doctor
- Penetrating injury to sole of foot – clean wound and give prophylactic antibiotics (see wounds page 136)

Crush injuries of the foot

- Often associated with significant swelling and pain
- Compartment syndrome is a complication
- If severe – discuss with a senior or orthopaedic doctor for admission for elevation and observation

Part C
INFANTS

General information	187
The unwell child	188
Abdominal problems	192
Breathlessness	196
CNS problems and injury	204
Injury	207

GENERAL INFORMATION

General information

Approximate weight (kg) = (age + 4) ×2
Fluid bolus = 20 ml/kg

Age (years)	Respiratory rate (breaths per minute)	Heart rate (beats per minute)	Systolic BP (mmHg)
<1	30–40	110–160	70–90
1–<2	25–35	100–150	80–95
2–<5	25–30	95–140	80–100
5–12	20–25	80–120	90–110
>12	15–20	60–100	100–120

Blood pressure (systolic)= 80+(age×2) mmHg
Capillary refill = normally 2 seconds or less after pressing on the sternum for 5 seconds

A **A**lert
V responds to **v**oice
P responds to **p**ain
U **U**nresponsive

Common drug doses

Paracetamol (Calpol): over 3 months first dose 20 mg/kg, subsequently 15 mg/kg
Ibuprofen: over 1 year 5 mg/kg
Morphine: (Oramorph): 250 mcg/kg
Benzylpenicillin: 50 mg/kg IV 4–6 hourly
Ceftriaxone: 80 mg/kg IV 6 hourly
Morphine IV: 0.1 mg/kg
Diazepam: 100–250 mcg/kg IV rectal 500 mcg/kg
Lorazepam: 0.1 mg/kg
Paraldehyde: 0.4 ml/kg rectal or IM
Glucose: 5ml/kg of 10% dextrose

INFANTS

The unwell child
The febrile child

Many children present with a fever but the focus of infection can be hard to find. A systematic examination will help not to miss anything. Listen to the parents, trust their intuition and your own. Get help early if you are concerned.

What to ask

- Onset of pyrexia and if any response to antipyretics
- Feeding – decreased fluid/diet intake
- Wet nappies – decreased urine output
- Unusually quiet, sleeping excessively
- Anybody else at home unwell

What to look for

Undress child and examine head to toe
- Assess AVPU (see page 187) – if not A – **Get help**
- If signs of shock/dehydration or meningism **Get help**
- Do not forget to examine the ears and the throat and look for rashes. If non-blanching see meningococcal disease (page 190–191)
- Most urine infections present with pyrexia

Investigations

These will depend on the clinical features
- Capillary blood glucose
- Urine analysis
- Swabs
- Discuss with senior or paediatrics the value of X-rays and blood samples

Management

- Antipyretics – paracetamol and ibuprofen
- Remove clothes
- Ensure a cool environment

THE UNWELL CHILD

Who needs referral

- If persisting pyrexia despite antipyretics
- Any child under 3 months
- Any child with unclear source of infection

Who can be sent home

- Children whose source of infection has been identified and can be safely treated at home
- Children whose temperature has come down with antipyretics
- Parents happy to take child home and are able to return if child deteriorates

INFANTS

Meningococcal disease

> **Suspect meningococcal disease if:**
> - Fever
> - Meningism or non-blanching rash
>
> Then give 80 mg/kg ceftriaxone and **Get help**

What to ask

- Onset of illness
- Feeding
- Vomiting
- Altered consciousness
- Convulsions
- Any rash

What to look for

- **Older child** (over 4 years): pyrexia, neck stiffness, photophobia, vomiting, headache, decreased or altered consciousness, convulsions
- **Younger child**: pyrexia, poor feeding, irritability, drowsy, bulging tense fontanelle, apnoea, convulsions
- RASH: expose the whole child!
  - purpuric/petechial, non-blanching
  - initially may be blanching or absent
- Prolonged capillary refill, tachycardic becoming bradycardic pre-terminally, tachypnoeic

> Neck stiffness is an unreliable sign in neonates and infants. Kernig's sign is unreliable in children

THE UNWELL CHILD

Investigations

- Blood capillary glucose
- FBC, U&E's, blood glucose, blood cultures, one clotted and one EDTA sample for meningitis antibodies and polymerase chain reaction (PCR)
- Swabs: nasopharyngeal, skin rash scraping. Can be taken once initial management completed

Other causes of meningism

- Pneumonia
- Subarachnoid haemorrhage
- Acute otitis media
- Severe tonsillitis
- Encephalitis

Management

Get help
- Oxygen
- IV access or intraosseous
- If signs of shock – prolonged capillary refill, tachycardic, hypotensive – give fluid bolus 20 ml/kg
- If fitting *see* status epilepticus (page 206)
- Lower pyrexia with paracetamol and/or ibuprofen

All patients must be admitted to the paediatrician

INFANTS

Abdominal problems
Abdominal pain/vomiting

What to ask

- Duration of symptoms
- If vomiting – frequency and nature – if 'projectile'
- Blood in stool – 'redcurrant jelly' in intussusception
- Symptoms of dehydration
  - Reduced urine output/dry nappies
  - Lethargy/sleepiness

What to look for

- Signs of significant dehydration – if present **Get help**
  - Lethargy / sleepiness
  - Tachycardia
  - Tachypnoea
  - Dry mucous membranes
  - Depressed fontanelle in infants
  - Prolonged capillary return
- Abdominal mass or tenderness
- Hernial orifices, scrotum and umbilicus for hernias

Investigations

- Capillary blood glucose
- If child has symptoms or signs of significant dehydration – FBC, U&E's, blood glucose
- Abdominal X-ray – if abdominal tenderness or mass

Management

- If there are any signs of significant dehydration give an IV fluid bolus of 20 ml/kg of 0.9% saline
- **Intussusception** – age 6 months to 4 years. Episodes of sudden screaming and drawing of legs up are typical. Blood in stool and abdominal mass are diagnostic. Refer all possible cases to a surgeon
- **Pyloric stenosis** – age 2–10 weeks. Repeated vomiting often projectile is typical. Abdominal mass may be felt during a test feed. Refer all possible cases to a surgeon

ABDOMINAL PROBLEMS

- **Appendicitis** – in children often an atypical presentation – have low threshold for referral to a surgeon
- **Hernias** – if irreducible or tender refer to a surgeon for further assessment

Other causes of abdominal pain in children include:

- Constipation
- Presentation of sickle cell disease
- Lower lobe pneumonia
- Testicular torsion
- Pregnancy

Diarrhoea and vomiting

What to ask

- Duration of symptoms
- Symptoms of dehydration
  - Reduced urine output/nappies drier than normal
  - Lethargy/sleepiness
- If keeping anything down – is child taking fluids
- Blood in stool

What to look for

- Signs of significant dehydration – if present **Get help**
  - Lethargy/sleepiness
  - Tachycardia
  - Tachypnoea
  - Dry mucous membranes
  - Depressed fontanelle in infants
  - Prolonged capillary return
- Abdominal tenderness/mass

Investigations

- Capillary blood glucose
- If child has symptoms or signs of significant dehydration – FBC, U&E's, blood glucose, blood cultures if pyrexial
- Stool sample

Management

- If there are any signs of significant dehydration give an IV fluid bolus of 20 ml/kg of 0.9% saline

Who needs referral

- Children under 3 months of age
- Children with signs or symptoms of significant dehydration
- Children with blood in stool
- Children whose parents aren't coping

ABDOMINAL PROBLEMS

If sending a child home

- Give parents advice to:
  - Return if child develops symptoms of significant dehydration
  - Give small volumes of fluids frequently

INFANTS

Breathlessness

Asthma

What to ask

- Chest tightness, wheeze, cough, shortness of breath
- Previous hospital/PICU admissions
- Nocturnal symptoms
- Increase in severity of symptoms
- Recent steroids/infection or GP visits

What to look for

	Moderate	Severe	Life-threatening
PEFR in over 5-year-olds only	>50%	33–50%	<33%
Respiratory rate (breaths/min)	<50: 2–5 years <30: over 5 years	>50: 2–5 years >30: over 5 years	Silent chest
Pulse (beats/min)	<130: 2–5 years <120: over 5 years	>130: 2–5 years >120: over 5 years	Bradycardia
Other features	No clinical features of severe asthma	Too breathless to talk or eat, accessory muscle use	Confusion, exhaustion, coma, **Get help**

Investigations

- Chest X-ray (not routinely needed for moderate asthma)
- ABG only if life-threatening

Management

- **Life-threatening and severe – Get help.**
  Commence high-flow oxygen and nebulised salbutamol 2–5 years: 2.5 mg; over 5 years: 5 mg

BREATHLESSNESS

- **Moderate** – 2–10 puffs of usual β_2 agonist, eg salbutamol, via spacer or facemask. Reassess after 15 minutes and if improving
  - Continue inhalers as needed up to 1 hourly and consider prednisolone 20 mg (2–5 years) or 30–40 mg (over 5 years) daily for 3 days. Ensure GP follow-up
- If not improving repeat inhaled β_2 agonist every 20–30 minutes, give prednisolone 20 mg (2–5 years) or 30–40 mg (over 5 years) and reassess: is this severe asthma?

Who needs referral

- Discuss all with senior or on-call paediatrician

INFANTS

INFANTS

Bronchiolitis

Rare after 1 year of age.

What to ask

- Runny nose usually prior to cough and breathlessness
- Reduced feeding (due to increasing difficulty in breathing), difficult to assess if breast fed
- Prematurity (increased risk of bronchiolitis if premature)

What to look for

- Tachypnoea
- Subcostal and intercostal recession
- Wheezes and/or crackles in chest
- Signs of significant dehydration – if present **Get help**
  - Lethargy/sleepiness
  - Tachycardia
  - Tachypnoea
  - Dry mucous membranes
  - Depressed fontanelle in infants
  - Prolonged capillary return

Investigations

- Pulse oximetry
- Chest X-ray if requiring admission (see below)

Management

- If low oxygen saturations, give oxygen by holding mask near to face or use head box
- IV fluids if there is significant dehydration

Who needs referral

- Low oxygen saturations
- Any difficulty in feeding, as can rapidly deteriorate
- Presentations late at night
- Worsening symptoms

If sending patient home

- Discuss with senior or on-call paediatrician
- Ensure parental understanding and ability to return if any deterioration
- Ensure GP follow-up

Croup

Normally affects age group 6 months to 6 years.

What to ask

- Duration of associated symptoms, usually will have had runny nose prior to attendance
- Gradual onset of severe barking cough
- Immunisation history
- Contacts with unwell children, eg at playgroup

What to look for

- Mild pyrexia
- If they look very unwell and are unable to swallow own saliva, consider acute epiglottitis and **Get help**, do not upset patient, eg cannulate or lie them down, as this may make things worse
- Recession, use of accessory muscles and stridor

Investigations

- Pulse oximetry – if less than 93% on air **Get help**

Management

- Ensure calm environment for child and parents
- Give either nebulised budesonide or oral dexamethasone according to local policy

Who needs referral

- Refer all but those with the mildest of symptoms
- Any child less than 12 months age
- Evening presentations as croup worsens at night

BREATHLESSNESS

If sending home ensure

- Parents understand need to return, and are able to return, if symptoms recur
- Follow-up with GP

My department's policy on treatment for croup is:

INFANTS

Upper respiratory tract infection

What to ask

- Duration and nature of symptoms, eg runny nose, cough, earache
- Contacts with unwell children, eg at playgroup
- Immunisation history

What to look for

- If they look very unwell and are unable to swallow own saliva, consider acute epiglottitis and **Get help,** do not upset patient, eg cannulate or lie them down, as this may make things worse
- Pyrexia
- Nasal discharge or blockage
- Red bulging tympanic membrane as in otitis media
- Inflamed throat or purulent exudate on tonsils
- Rash

Investigations

- Swabs of inflamed throat with follow-up of results as local protocol, eg copy to GP

Management

- Simple coryzal symptoms require reassurance and advice to use paracetamol and/or ibuprofen (if no contraindications) to relieve symptoms
- Antibiotics are occasionally indicated in inflamed throats but check local policy regards awaiting swab results
- Otitis media is treated with adequate analgesia and antibiotics as local policy

BREATHLESSNESS

Who needs referral

- Refer if pyrexial with unclear focus of infection or >38°C despite antipyretic therapy

If sending patient home

- Ensure parental understanding and ability to return if any deterioration
- Ensure GP follow-up

My department's policy on antibiotic treatment for otitis media:

INFANTS

CNS problems and injury

Convulsions

If patient currently fitting go to status epilepticus (page 206)

What to ask

- First seizure
- Recent illness, pyrexia
- Character and duration of seizure
- Recent head injury
- Family history
- If known epileptic ask about current medication and frequency of fits

What to look for

- AVPU (see page 187) if not Alert **Get help**
- Injury as a result or as a cause of seizure
- Source of infection (check chest, ears, mouth)
- Rash – non-blanching (see Meningococcal disease page 190–191)
- Pyrexia
- Signs of shock: prolonged capillary refill, tachycardia, hypotensive – **Get help**

Investigations

- Capillary blood glucose
- FBC, U&E's, blood glucose, blood cultures if pyrexial
- Urine analysis

Management

- Place in the recovery position
- Oxygen
- Treat a low capillary blood glucose with 5 ml/kg of 10% dextrose IV

CNS PROBLEMS AND INJURY

- Rectal temperature, if pyrexial give paracetamol 20 mg/kg

Find time to reassure parents and explain what has happened

Who needs referral

- Febrile convulsions that can be sent home: if pyrexia has settled/not first fit/if parents happy to take child home
- Known epileptic patients that can be sent home: no neurological deficit/no underlying infection/not a recent increase in the number of fits/parents happy to take child home
- If pyrexial not settled
- First fits
- Parents unhappy to take child home
- Underlying infection
- Recent increase in frequency of fits
- Parents unhappy to take child home

Status epilepticus
Status epilepticus flowchart – Get help

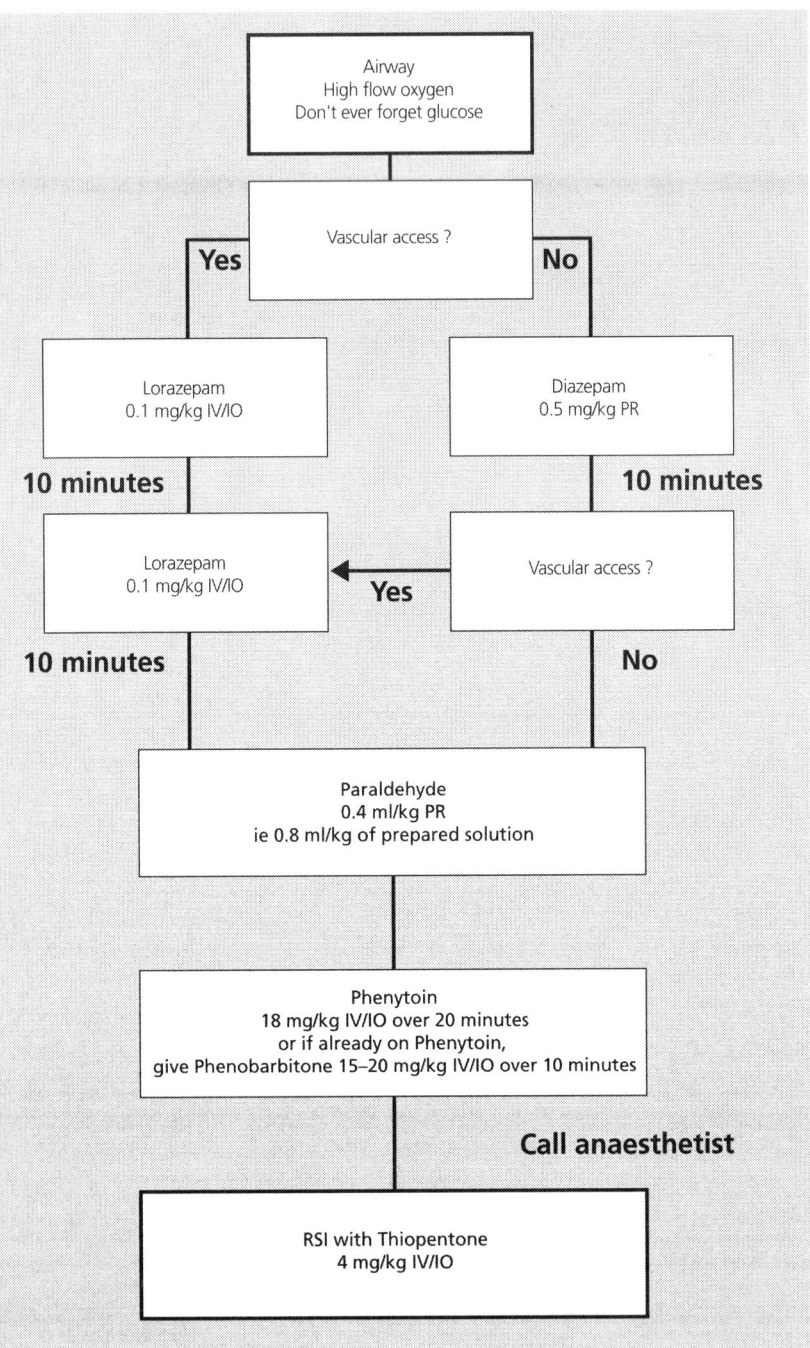

```
                    ┌─────────────────────────┐
                    │         Airway          │
                    │    High flow oxygen     │
                    │ Don't ever forget glucose│
                    └───────────┬─────────────┘
                                │
                    ┌───────────┴─────────────┐
              Yes   │    Vascular access ?    │   No
           ┌────────┤                         ├────────┐
           │        └─────────────────────────┘        │
           │                                           │
  ┌────────┴────────┐                        ┌─────────┴────────┐
  │   Lorazepam     │                        │    Diazepam      │
  │ 0.1 mg/kg IV/IO │                        │  0.5 mg/kg PR    │
  └─────────────────┘                        └──────────────────┘
**10 minutes**                                      **10 minutes**
           │                                           │
  ┌────────┴────────┐          Yes          ┌──────────┴───────┐
  │   Lorazepam     │◄──────────────────────┤ Vascular access ?│
  │ 0.1 mg/kg IV/IO │                       │                  │
  └─────────────────┘                       └──────────────────┘
**10 minutes**                                         No
           │                                           │
           └─────────────────┬─────────────────────────┘
                             │
              ┌──────────────┴──────────────────┐
              │        Paraldehyde              │
              │       0.4 ml/kg PR              │
              │ ie 0.8 ml/kg of prepared solution│
              └──────────────┬──────────────────┘
                             │
         ┌───────────────────┴─────────────────────────┐
         │                Phenytoin                    │
         │      18 mg/kg IV/IO over 20 minutes         │
         │        or if already on Phenytoin,          │
         │ give Phenobarbitone 15–20 mg/kg IV/IO over 10 minutes│
         └───────────────────┬─────────────────────────┘
                             │                **Call anaesthetist**
              ┌──────────────┴──────────────┐
              │     RSI with Thiopentone    │
              │       4 mg/kg IV/IO         │
              └─────────────────────────────┘
```

Injury

Head injury

What to ask

- Mechanism of injury
- Witnessed loss of consciousness
- Whether vomited and how many times
- Past history of fits or coagulation problems

What to look for

- Behaviour of child
- Local tenderness, swelling and bruising
- Consider whether appearance of injury is consistent with history
- Calculate the child's GCS (*see* inside back cover)
  - If less than 15 – **Get help**
- Temperature – co-existing illness may make children vomit or seem drowsy

Investigations

- X-ray or CT scan – find out your department's policy for further investigation of head injuries

Management

- If the child seems quiet ensure they have adequate analgesia – and reassess them in 30 minutes

Who needs referral

- Find out your department's policy for admission of children after head injury

If sending a child home

- Explain head injury instructions to the parents

INFANTS

Limping

What to ask

- Any history of injury – if yes see limb injuries (page 210–211)
- Systemic upset – pyrexia, vomiting, etc.
- Recent viral illness
- Previous problems/other joint problems

What to look for

- Systemic signs – pyrexia, tachycardia
- Whole of lower body from back to toes
- Try to identify side causing problem – watch the child walking
- Any apparent tenderness, rash, erythema, local warmth, swelling or bruising
- Move all joints in all directions

Investigations

- FBC, ESR, blood cultures if:
  - Any systemic signs or symptoms
  - Any areas of erythema or local warmth
- X-ray or ultrasound (find out your department's policy) – if any signs or symptoms indicating a specific area

Management

- Analgesia if in pain and antipyretic if pyrexial

Who needs referral

- If systemic signs or symptoms
- If unable to exclude a septic arthritis (see page 122)
- If unable to weight bear/severe pain
- Refer these patients to an orthopaedic doctor

If sending a child home

- Check your department's policy for the follow-up of a limping child

INJURY

Hip – causes of a limp

Irritable hip – transient synovitis of the hip. Age 1–10. Systemically well with normal X-ray and limp that settles within a few days
- **Perthes disease** – avascular necrosis of femoral head. Age 3–11 with flattening of femoral head seen on X-ray
- **Slipped femoral epiphysis** – usually older child (10–15 years). X-ray including lateral view shows slip of epiphyseal plate
- **Septic arthritis** – *see* septic arthritis (page 122)

Limb injuries

What to ask

- Mechanism of injury – check consistent with injury
- Previous injuries/problems

What to look for

- Children can be difficult to examine:
  - Be sympathetic, patient and methodical
  - Examination may be much easier once appropriate analgesia has been given
- Check for tenderness/swelling/bruising/local warmth

Investigations

- Have a low threshold for X-ray if the history is vague or the examination is inconsistent or incomplete
- Greenstick fractures (buckling of the bone) can occur due to the relative softness of the bone. Trace round the cortex of the bone looking for irregularity and angulation
- Epiphyses add to the complexity of X-ray interpretation – discuss with a senior or orthopaedic doctor if unsure
- If X-ray equivocal treat as fracture

Management

- Ensure adequate analgesia has been given
- For most injuries see appropriate page in Injury

Specific children's limb problems

Pulled elbow
- Pulling injury to arm in under 6-year-olds
- Pronated arm held limply at side with **no** tenderness swelling or bruising. X-ray the elbow if in doubt
- To reduce the elbow:
  - Explain what you are doing and warn that the child will cry
  - Supinate the arm until a click is felt at elbow
  - Child will be better within 15 minutes, if not discuss with senior or orthopaedic doctor

Supracondylar fracture of the elbow
- Fall onto arm with swollen tender elbow
- Check wrist pulses as injury to brachial artery can occur
- X-ray can be difficult to interpret – get help if unsure
- Find out your department's policy for this injury

Toddler's fracture
- Often minor fall with lower tibial tenderness or swelling
- Undisplaced fracture of the lower tibia which may not initially be apparent on the X-ray
- If fracture seen or suspected on examination – discuss with a senior or orthopaedic doctor

INFANTS

Burns

What to ask

- Mechanism of burn – heat source, duration of exposure
- If fire – whether significant exposure to smoke
  - Hoarseness of the voice or stridor
  - Singeing of facial hair
  - Soot in the nostrils
  If any of these are present – **Get help**

What to look for

- Location and depth of burn. Use Lund & Browder chart to measure and record size.
- If burn or smoke inhalation involves airway – **Get help**
- Consider if burn appearance is consistent with history
- Temperature – children quickly become hypothermic particularly if covered in cold, wet towels

Investigations

- Capillary blood glucose
- If giving IV fluid/analgesia – FBC, U&E's, blood glucose
- Carboxyhaemoglobin level if significant exposure to smoke – take a venous or capillary sample if ABGs aren't needed

Management

- Adequate analgesia – may need IV morphine. Don't forget simple measures such as covering the burn
- IV fluid if the burn is over 10% of body surface area – find out your department's policy for IV fluids in burns
- Dressings – find out your department's policy

INJURY

Who needs referral

- Any burn of greater than 10% size
- Smoke inhalation or any airway burn
- Any full thickness burn
- If inconsistency between history and examination
- Any burn involving :
  - The genitalia, perineum or buttocks
  - The neck
  - Any hand burn over a joint

If you are sending a child home

- Ensure arrangements are made for follow-up according to your departmental policy

INFANTS

Child abuse

> If you are suspicious of any form of child abuse DO NOT confront the parents – discuss with a senior or a paediatrician

Neglect

- The commonest form of child abuse encountered in the Emergency department
- Indicators include:
  - Preventable accidents, eg. children falling down stairs with no stair-gate
  - Lack of hygiene
  - Poor interaction between parent and child, eg disinterest/inappropriate language such as swear words
  - Delay in seeking help
- Accident prevention advice and/or health visitor referral may be all that is required

Physical forms of abuse

- There are very few physical injuries that are diagnostic of child abuse
- Take extreme care to ensure there is no other explanation for the injury
- Factors which should alert to the possibility of abuse include:
  - Multiple attendances
  - Discrepancy between history/mechanism of injury and physical findings
  - Injuries in non-mobile children
- Some injuries which may cause confusion:
  - Torn lip frenulum – usually entirely accidental from fall onto face
  - Cigarette burn – impetigo may have a similar appearance
  - Spiral limb fractures – can occur entirely accidentally

Management

- If you have any cause for concern always discuss with a senior or a paediatrician
- Find out your department's policy for dealing with possible child abuse

INDEX

This index concentrates on conditions and symptoms. Page numbers in **bold type** indicate the most comprehensive or important treatment of the subject. In other words, start there.

abbreviations   xiii
abdominal injury   158, **170–1**, 174
abdominal mass   89, 107
abdominal pain   48, 74, **88**, 89–102, **103–4**
   child   **192–3**
   gynaecological   115, 116, 118
   haematemesis and/or melaena   107, 109
ABG (arterial blood gases)   xvi, **21**, 24, **32**
abscess   46, **110**, 140
N-acetylcysteine (NAC) use   64, **65**
Achilles tendon injury   178–9, 180–1
acromioclavicular joint injury   160, 161
acute coronary syndrome   5, **6–7**, 88
acute heart failure   12, 13, 16
adenosine use   **15**
adrenaline, resistance to   69
AF (atrial fibrillation)   12, **16**, 36, 105
aggressive behaviour   ix, 53, 54, 76, 79
agitated patient   24, **79–80**
AIDS *see* HIV infection
airway compromised   130, 134–5
alcohol   ix, 53, 126
   abuse   34, **81–2**, 92, 103, 109
   fit/epilepsy and   40
   with overdose   62, 64
   painful joints and   120
allergic reaction   **69**, 143
AMPLE mnemonic   130
amylase levels   88, 92, **93**
anaesthetic, local   **138**
anal fissure   107
analgesia   **xi-xii,** 138
angina   5, **6–7**

INDEX

angioedema   69
animal bites   137, 139, 140, 143
ankle   120, **180–1**, 182
ankylosing spondylitis   154, 172
anticoagulants
   arterial occlusion   105
   haematemesis/melaena   107, 109
   headache and   36, 57, 146, 147
aortic aneurysm   88, **89**, 101, 106, 123
aortic stenosis   **42**
appendicitis   51, 88, **99–100**, 116
   child   193
arm   **164–5**
   child   **210–11**, 214
arterial blood gases (ABG)   xvi, **21**, 24, **32**
arterial occlusion, acute   **105–6**
arthritis   119, 122, 125, **125**, 154
   septic   119, **122**, 125, 140
      child   209
aspirin   32, 105, 120
assault   **128–9**, 143, 148, 169
asthma   19, **20–1**, 22
   child   **196–7**
atrial fibrillation (AF)   12, **16**, 36, 105
aura/prodrome   38, 56, 58
AVPU scale   34, **35**, **187**, 188

back injury   **172–3**
back pain   48, 89, 90, 94, **123–4**
backache, pregnancy and   115, 118
balance disturbed   36, 146
bee/wasp sting   69
Bennett's fracture   169
beta-blockers, adrenaline resistance and   69
biochemical values   **xv-xvi**
bites   **143**, 169
   animal   137, 139, 140
   human   129, 137, 139, 140
   insect   52, 69, 122, 143
bladder distention   79
blood gases, normal values   **xvi**
bone pain   74

INDEX

bowel sounds   90, 102
breathing
   asymmetrical   19, 134
   in major trauma   130
breathlessness   **19, 32**
   allergic reaction   69
   chest injury   158
   chest pain and   10, 22, 26, 30
   child   **196–201**
   cough/sputum and   22, 24
   faint and   38
   nocturnal   20, 30, 196, 200
   sounds absent   28
   see also tachypnoea
broad complex tachycardia   12, **13**
bronchiolitis   **198–9**
burns   46, **132–3**
   child   132, **212–13**
   depth/size   132

C-spine   130, 146, 154–5
CAGE mnemonic   **81**
cancer *see* malignancy
capillary refill prolonged   **44**
   see also shock
carbon monoxide poisoning   **61**
cardiac, *see also* heart
cardiac arrest   **4**
cardiac chest pain   **5, 6**, 8, 11
cardiac syncope   **42**
cardiac tamponade   4, 10
cardiomyopathy   **42**
cardiovascular problems   32, 33, 105
   see also aortic aneurysm; atrial fibrillation (AF); myocardial infarction (MI)
carotid bruit   36
cauda equina syndrome   123
cerebrovascular accident (CVA)   33, **36–7**
cervical spine   130, 146, 154–6
chest drain insertion   **29**
chest infection   19, **22–3**, 43
   child   **202–3**

INDEX

chest injury   19, 28, **158–9**
chest pain   **5, 11**
   breathlessness and   20, 22, 26, 28, 30
   cardiac   5, 6–11
   faint and   38
   palpitation and   13
   in sickle cell disease   74
chest sounds   24, 28
   crackles   6, 16, 19, 22, 30
     in child   198
   see also wheeze
child   **187**
   abdominal pain   **192–3**
   abuse of   **214–15**
   back pain   123
   breathlessness   196–203
   burns   132, 214
   convulsions   204–6
   diarrhoea and vomiting   **194–5**
   drug doses   **187**
   epididymo-orchitis   113
   febrile   **188–9**, 204, 205
   Glasgow coma scale *see* **inside back cover**
   meningococcal disease   **190–1**
   painful joints   125
   testicular torsion   **112**
   vomiting   192–5
cholecystitis   88, 93, **94–5**
chronic obstructive pulmonary disease (COPD)   19, 22, **24–5**, 29
clavicle fracture   160
cluster headache   **61**
colchicine, precautions   121
collapse   28, **33**, **42**
Colles' fracture   166
coma   68
   AVPU scale   34, **35**, **187**, 188
   Glasgow coma scale
     adult: **inside front cover**   34, 36
     child: **inside back cover**   207
communication difficulties   ix
compartment syndrome   **165**, 183

INDEX

complaints procedure   ix
confidentiality   ix
confused patients   ix, 22, 24
conjunctival redness   84, **85**
consciousness reduced   30, **33**, 34, 36
   assault and   128
   diabetes   53, 54
   drug overdose   66
   faint   38
   head injury and   146, 207
   headache and   56
   palpitations and   14
   rash and   190
   see also collapse; coma; epilepsy; faint; fit
constipation   51, 90
   child   193
contact lens lost   85
contraceptives   26, 36, 70, 116
convulsions   **33**, 38, 68, 74
   child   **204–5**
   rash and   190
   see also epilepsy
COPD (chronic obstructive pulmonary disease)   19, 22, **24–5**, 29
corneal ulceration   84, **85**
costochondritis   11
cough   20, 22, 46, 69
   child   198, 200, 202
   haemoptysis   22, 26, 158
croup   **200–1**
cruciate ligament injury   176, 177
crush injury   139
   foot   182, **183**
   hand   168, 169
CURB mnemonic   **22**
CVA (cerebrovascular accident)   33, **36–7**

deep vein thrombosis (DVT)   **70–1**, 106
defecation, pain on   107
dehydration
   abdominal pain and   50, 90, 99
   child   188, 192, 194, 198

dehydration (*continued*)
   collapse and   33
   joint pain and   120
delirium tremens   **81**
dental complaints   148, **150–1**
diabetes   34, **53–5**, 105
   ketoacidosis   32, **54–5**, 104
   soft tissue infections   46, 110, 140
   stroke and   36
diarrhoea and vomiting   46, 50, 107
   child   **194–5**
digoxin, therapeutic levels   xvi
diuretics   30, 101, 120
diverticulitis   88, **96**
documentation of injuries   126, 148, 168
domestic violence   126–7
drug abuse   34, 40, 79
   ecstasy   52
   injection sites   46, 52, 66
drug overdose   **62–3**
   co-proxamol   66
   opiate   34, **66–7**
   paracetamol   **64–5**
   tricyclic antidepressant   **68**
drugs (medicinal)
   change of   38
   child's dosage   **187**
   see also under individual drug or type (eg aspirin, oral contraceptives *etc*)
DVT (deep vein thrombosis)   **70–1**, 106
dysphagia   134–5, 200, 202
dyspnoea *see* breathlessness
dysuria *see* urinary symptoms

ear problems   146, 191, 202
ectopic pregnancy   88, 93, **116–17**
elbow injury   **162–3**, 163, 164
   child   211
elderly person
   back pain/injury   123, 172
   bladder distention   79
   hip fracture   174–5

hypothermia   72–3
knee injury   177
neck injury   156
painful joints   122
electrocardiogram (ECG)   **11**
  ectopic beats   12, 18
  palpitations and   **12**, 13, 14, 16
emergency department working risks   ix
encephalitis   56, 191
endocrinology, normal values   **xv**
epicondyle fracture   162, 163
epididymo-orchitis   **113–14**
epiglottitis   200, 202
epilepsy   34, **40–1**, 79, 81
  child   204–5, **206**
  status epilepticus   **206**
erythema   46, 69, 140, 143
exercise
  sudden headache and   57
  tolerance decreased   24, 28
external meatus, blood at   174
eye
  conjunctival redness   84, **85**, 148
  injury   **152–3**
  movement   36, 146
  painful   **84–5**
  papilloedema   60
  peri-orbital haematoma   146
  pupil size   62
    dilated   68
  fixed   84
  pinpoint   34, 66
  retinal changes   57, 84
  symptoms, painful joints and   119
  see also vision

F's guide to gallstones   **94**
face   **148–9**, 150
  local anaesthesia   138
  see also ear; eye; mouth; nose
faint (vasovagal syncope)   **38–9**
fall from height   154, 174, 182

INDEX

fall onto outstretched hand (FOOSH)   162, 164, 166
fatty meal eaten recently   88, 94
febrile convulsions   204, 205
feet *see* foot
female patient
   gallstones   94
   menstruating   46, 97
   pelvic inflammatory disease   97
   see also contraceptives; hormone replacement therapy
      (HRT); pregnancy
femoral pulses weak/absent   89
femur injury   174–5, 209
fever *see* pyrexia
fibula fracture   **178**
finger injury   168, 169
fit   33, **40–1**
   diabetic   53, 54
   headache/head injury   56, 146
flail segment   **158**
fontanelle   190, 194, 198
food intake
   fatty   88, 94
   lack of   38
   protein   120
FOOSH (fall onto outstretched hand)   162, 164, 166
foot
   injury   181, **182–3**
   local anaesthesia   138
   painful/swollen   74, 120
foreign body
   in eye   152, 153
   swallowed/inhaled   **134–5**
   in wound   136, 138
foreign travel   22, 24, 52, 70
fracture
   greenstick   210
   open   137
   spiral limb   214
   stress   182
   see also under the limb or joint affected

Galeazzi fracture   163

INDEX

gallstones 92, 94
gastrocnemius injury 178
gastrointestinal problems
  bleeding 107
  child 192–5
  gastroenteritis 43, **50–1**, 104, 107
  irritable bowel syndrome 104
  obstruction 51, 88, **90–1**, 93
  painful joints and 119
  perforation 88, **102**
GCS *see* Glasgow coma scale (GCS)
genitalia *see* testicles; vagina
giant cell arteritis **60**
Glasgow coma scale (GCS): **inside front cover** 34, 56
  child: **inside back cover** 207
glaucoma 84
glyceryl trinitrate (GTN) infusion **31**
gout 119, **120–1**, 125
greenstick fracture 210

haemarthrosis 176
haematemesis 50, **109**
haematological values **xv**
haematuria 49, 101
haemoptysis 22, 26, 158
haemorrhage 33, 131, 136
haemorrhoids 107
hallucinations 76, 81
hand 74, **168–9**, 213
  local anaesthesia 138
head injury **146–7**, 148, 150
  agitation and 79, 81
  child 204, **207**
  fitting/unconscious 34, 40
headache 36, **56**, 57, **60–1**, 146
  early morning 60, 61
  rash and 44, 190
heart
  failure 12, 13, 16, **30–1**
  ischaemic heart disease 11, 36, **42**, 88
  murmur 10, 30, 105
  see also cardiac

INDEX

heart beat
  arrhythmias   6, 68
  rate raised   13, 14, 16
  regularity   12, 13, 14
heat stroke/heat exhaustion   52
heel, injury   178
help, when to ask for   vii
hepatitis B   125, 142, 143
hernia   90
  child   193
hip   120, 125, **174–5**
  child   **208–9**
HIV infection   22, 64
  injury/bite   142, 143
Homan's sign   **70**
HONK (hyperosmolar non-ketotic hyperglycaemia)   **54–5**
hormone replacement therapy (HRT)   26, 70
how to use this book   vii-viii
human bites   129, 137, 140, 143
humeral head/neck fracture   160
hydrocele   112
hyperglycaemia   **54–5**, 79
hyperosmolar non-ketotic hyperglycaemia (HONK)   **54–5**
hypertension, headache and   36, 56, 60
hyperventilation   19, 32
hyphaema   152, 153
hypoglycaemia   34, **53**, 79, 81
hypotension
  chest pain and   6, 10, 22
  palpitation and   12, 13
  postural   38, **42**
hypothermia   4, **72–3**
  child   212
hypoxia   4, **24**, 79

immobility   26, 70
immunocompromised patient   52, 110
  painful joints   46, 122, 125
incontinence   33, 38
indigestion, chest pain   11
infant *see* child
infection   **43**, **52**

INDEX

agitation/alcohol and   79, 81
painful joints and   125
septic shock   43, **46–7**
see also septic arthritis
inflammatory bowel disease   51, 102, 107, 110
inhaled foreign body   **134–5**
insect bites   52, 69, 122, 143
intestinal see gastrointestinal
intoxicated patient see alcohol; drug abuse; drug overdose
intracranial pressure raised   **61**
intravenous analgesia   **xii**
intravenous drug abusers (IVDAs) see drug abuse
intussusception   192
irritable bowel syndrome   104
irritable hip   209
ischaemic heart disease   11, 36, **42**, 88
IVDAs (intravenous drug abusers) see drug abuse

jaundice   92
jaw, mandibular injury   150
joint   **119**, **125**
   artificial/replaced   122
   aspiration   120
   effusion/haemarthrosis   176
   pain (generalised)   46, 60, **119**, 120, 140
   see also arthritis; individual joint

Kernig's sign   **44**, 190
ketoacidosis, diabetic   32, **54–5**, 104
knee   120, 122, 125, **176–7**

left ventricular failure (LVF)   **30–1**
leg   70, **178–9**
   child   **208–11**, 214
limp
   child   **208–9**
   intermittent claudication   105
lithium, therapeutic levels   xvi
liver complaints   64, 109
local anaesthetic   **138**
loss of consciousness see collapse; coma;
   consciousness reduced; epilepsy; faint; fit

lung disease *see* chest sounds; pneumonia/pneumothorax, pulmonary conditions
LVF (left ventricular failure) **30–1**
Lyme disease   122

major trauma   **130–1**, 172, 174
malaria   52
malignancy   22, 26, 52, 70, 123
   gastrointestinal   102, 103–4
malignant hypertension   60
Mallory Weiss tear   109
melaena   50, 96, **107–8**, **109**
   child   192
meningococcal disease   **44–5**, **190–1**
   differentiation   36, 40, 43, 56, 60
menstruating woman   46, 97
mental state altered   16, 46, 50
   see also alcohol; consciousness reduced; drug abuse
mental state health examination   **76–7**, 83
metabolic disorder   4, 32, 52, 79
migraine   56, 57, **58–9**
miscarriage   **115**, 116, **118**
Monteggia fracture   162
morphine, IV analgesia   **xii**
mouth
   dry   68
   injury   148, 214
Murphy's sign   **94**
myocardial infarction (MI)   5, **8–9**, 11, **42**, 88, 103

NAC (*N*-acetylcysteine) use   64, **65**
nails, injury to   169
narrow complex tachycardia   12, **14**
nausea and vomiting
   abdominal pain   94
   allergic reaction   69
   headache/head injury   44, 146
   testicular torsion   112
   urinary tract infection   49
neck
   burns   213
   injury   **154–6**, 160

INDEX

stiffness   43, 44, 56, 61, 190
needle thoracocentesis   **29**
needlestick injury   **142**
nerve damage   136, 168
neurological symptoms   32, 33, 36, 60, 123
nitrate-induced symptoms   38, **61**
non-Q-wave infarcts   **6–7**
nose   **149**
NSAIDs   103, 107, 109

oesophageal complaints   5, 107, 109
olecranon problems   162, 163
oral contraceptives   26, 36, 70, 116
orthstatic hypotension   38, **42**
osteoarthritis   119, **125**
otitis media   191, 202
Ottowa knee rules   176, **177**
ovarian cyst   116
overdose *see* drug overdose

P's guide to arterial occlusion   **105**
pain relief   **xi-xii, 138**
palpitations   **12**, 16, **18**, 38
pancreatitis   81, 88, **92–3**, 123
patella, injury/dislocation   176–7
peak expiry flow rate (PEFR)   20
pelvic inflammatory disease (PID)   88, **97–8**, 116
pelvis   **174–5**
penis   74, 174
   local anaesthesia   138
peptic ulcer disease   88, 93, 102, 103, 107
perianal abscess   **110**
pericarditis   5, **10**
peritonism   50, 88, 118
Perthes disease   209
photophobia   43, 44, 190
PID (pelvic inflammatory disease)   88, **97–8**, 116
pleural rub   26
pneumonia   5, 104, 191, 193
pneumothorax   5, 19, **28–9**, 158
poisoning   **62–3**
police report   126–7, 148, 168

postural hypotension   33, 38, **42**
pregnancy
    abdominal injury   **171**
    abdominal pain   70, 193
    ectopic   88, 93, **116–17**
    miscarriage   **115**, 116, **118**
    sickle cell disease and   74
    thromboembolism   26, 103
prolonged capillary refill   **44**
    see also shock
prostatitis   113
pseudogout   125
psychiatric conditions   76–82
pulmonary embolus (PE)   5, 11, 19, **26–7**
pulmonary oedema   13, 19, **30–1**
pulse rate in asthma   20
pupil size   62
    dilated   68
    fixed   84
    pinpoint   34, 66
pyloric stenosis   192
pyrexia   **43**, **52**
    abdominal pain and   50, 94, 96, 101, 102
    child   188–9, 204, 205, 207
    headache and   56, 60
    in septic shock   46
    sickle cell disease   74
    soft tissue infection   140
    testicular torsion   112

quadriceps muscle rupture   177

radial pulse deficit   164, 166
radio femoral delay   89
radius, fracture   162, 164, 166
rash   43, 46, 56, 60
    child   188, 214
    non-blanching   44, **190**, 204
    see also erythema
reactive arthritis   119
rectal complaints   **107–8**, 110
    see also melaena

INDEX

refusal of treatment **83**
Reiter's syndrome 125
renal disease 88, 89, **101**
   joint/back pain 120, 123
repetitive strain 166
respiratory depression 66
respiratory rate increased 20, 22
respiratory tract infection see chest infection
retinal changes 57, 84
rheumatic fever 125
rheumatoid arthritis 122, 125, 154
road traffic accident (RTA) 170, 172, 174
   neck injury 154, 156, 157
rotator cuff rupture 160, 161

S's guide to injury/wounds 129
salivation 134, 200, 202
SCA (sickle cell disease/anaemia) 52, **74–5**, 104, 125
   child 193
scaphoid injury 166
scrotum, pain/swelling 112, 113
seizure **40–1**
self-harm 62–8, **78**
septic arthritis 119, **122**, 125, 140, 163
   child 209
septic shock 43, **46–7**
sexual activity, headache and 57
sexually transmitted diseases 97–8, 113–14, 122
shaking/jerking see convulsions
shivering 72–3
shock
   abdominal pain 89, 92, 96, 97, 102
   abdominal/pelvic injury 170, 174
   allergic reaction 69, 143
   arteriovascular/bleeding disorders 105, 106, 107, 109
   atrial fibrillation 16
   chest pain/injury 8, 26, 30, 158
   child 188
   diabetes and 54
   emotional 38
   infection and 43, 50, 52
   pregnancy and 116, 118

shock (*continued*)
   septic **46–7**
   in sickle cell disease 74
   unconsciousness and 34
   urinary infection 49
shoulder **160–1**
   pain radiating to 116
sickle cell disease/anaemia (SCA) 52, **74–5**, 104, 125
   child 193
Simmond's test **178**
sinus disease 60
skull fracture 146
Smith's fracture 167
smoke inhalation 212, 213
smoking 22, 36
soft tissue infection 43, 137, **140–1**, 143
soft tissue injury 161, 169, 177, 181
speech
   breathlessness and 20, 30
      mental disorder and 76
spider naevi 92
spontaneous pneumothorax **28–9**
sputum 22, 24, 30
status epilepticus **206**
steroid use 46, 107, 110, 140
Stokes Adams attack **42**
stool *see* constipation; melaena
stress fracture 182
stress headache 56
stroke 33, 34, **36–7**, 79
subarachnoid haemorrhage 36, 56, **57**, 191
suicidal patients 62–8, 76, **78**
supracondylar fracture, child 211
suturing wounds **138–9**
swallowing difficulty 134–5, 200, 202
sweating 6, 8, 30, 53
   nocturnal 123
swelling
   joints *see* individual joint
   soft tissue 143

tachycardia 22, 26, 28

INDEX

broad complex   12, **13**
  child   194, 198
  narrow complex   12, **14**
  see also shock
tachypnoea   24, 26, 29, 72–3
  child   194, 198
  see also breathlessness
teeth   143, **150–1**
tendon damage   136, 168, 169
tenosynovitis   167
tension pneumothorax   4, **28–9**
tension-type headache   56
testicles
  burns to   213
  pain in   101, **111**, 112–14
  swollen   113
  torsion   **112**, 193
tetanus immunisation   **144–5**
thigh   **174–5**
thoracocentesis, needle   **29**
throat, sore, in child   200, 202
thromboembolism   4, **70–1**
thumb injury   166, 168
TIA (transient ischaemic attack)   33, **36–7**
tibial fracture   178
  child   211
toddler's fracture   211
toe injury   **182–3**
tongue bitten   33, 38
transient ischaemic attack (TIA)   33, **36–7**
trauma, major   **130–1**
treatment, refusal of   **83**
tuberculosis   52, 122

ulna   162–3, 164, 166
unconscious patient   **34–5**
ureteric colic   88, **101**
urethral discharge   113, 122, 174
urinary symptoms
  haematuria   49, 101
  infection (UTI)   43, **48–9**, 88, 101
  painful joints and   119

INDEX

urinary symptoms (*continued*)
    scrotal pain and   112, 113
    septic shock and   46

vagina
    bleeding   115, 118
    discharge   88, 97, 122
    pain in   101
vascular disorders   105–6
vasovagal syncope (faint)   33, **38–9**
violence   **128–9**, 143, 148, 169
vision   **84–5**
    aura   56, 58
    blurred   53, 68
    disturbed, with headache/head injury   60, 146, 148
    visual acuity   84, **152**
    see also eye
vomiting
    abdominal pain and   90, 94, 99
    child   **192–5**
    diabetes and   53
    haematemesis   50, **109**
    head injury and   207
    projectile   192
    see also diarrhoea and vomiting; nausea and vomiting

warfarin use   105, 107, 109
    see also anticoagulants
welding arc eye   **85**
wheeze   19, 20, **21**, 24, 30
    child   196, 198
wounds   **136–9**
    dirty   136, 139, 140–1, 144–5
wrist   125, **164–5**, 168

X-rays, cervical spine   154–5

Contact numbers

Emergency Department

Reception: ....
Resuscitation: ....
Majors: ....
Minors: ....

Doctors

Medical SHO: ....
Medical Registrar: ....
Medical assessment: ....
Surgical SHO: ....
Surgical Registrar: ....
Surgical assessment: ....
Urology: ....
Paediatric SHO: ....
Paediatric Registrar: ....
Orthopaedics SHO: ....
Obstetrics and Gynaecology SHO: ....
Plastics SHO: ....
ENT SHO: ....
Maxillary facial SHO: ....
Anaesthetist SHO: ....
Anaesthetic Registrar: ....
Intensive Care SHO: ....

Departments

Radiology ....
Pharmacy ....
Biochemistry ....
Haematology ....

PasTest

PasTest has been established since 1972 and is the leading provider of exam-related medical revision course sand books in the UK. The company has a dedicated customer services team to ensure that doctors can easily get up to date information about our products and to ensure that their orders are dealt with efficiently. Our extensive experience means that we are always one step ahead when it comes to knowledge of the current trends and contents of the Royal College exams.

In the last 12 months we have sold over 67,000 books to medical students and qualified doctors. These may be purchased through bookshops, over the telephone or online at our website. All books are reviewed prior to publication to ensure that they mirror the needs of candidates and therefore act as an invaluable aid to exam preparation.

Test yourself online
PasTest Online is a new database that will be launched this year. With more than 1500 Best of Five questions prepared by experts, PasTest Online:

- enables you to test yourself whenever you want
- is accessible whatever time of day
- is reasonably priced and has excellent exam revision tips
- has a choice of mock exam, random questions and specialist questions. This means that you can test yourself in certain weak areas or take a mock exam.

Interested? Try a free demo at www.pastestonline.co.uk

100% Money Back Guarantee
We're sure you will find our study books invaluable, but in the unlikely event that you are not entirely happy, we will give you your money back – guaranteed.

Delivery to your Door
With a busy lifestyle, nobody enjoys walking to the shops for something that may or may not be in stock. Let us take the hassle and deliver direct to your door. We will despatch your book within 24 hours of receiving your order. We also offer free delivery on books for medical students to UK addresses.

How to Order
www.pastest.co.uk
To order books safely and securely online, shop at our website.

Telephone: +44 (0)1565 752000
Have your credit card to hand when you call.

+44 (0) 1565 650264
Fax your order with your debit or credit card details.

PasTest Ltd, FREEPOST, Knutsford, Cheshire WA16 7BR
Send your order with your cheque (made payable to PasTest Ltd) and debit or credit card details to the above address. (Please complete your address details on the reverse of the cheque.)

Notes